The Woman's Yoga Book

The Woman's Yoga Book

ASANA AND PRANAYAMA

FOR ALL PHASES OF THE MENSTRUAL CYCLE

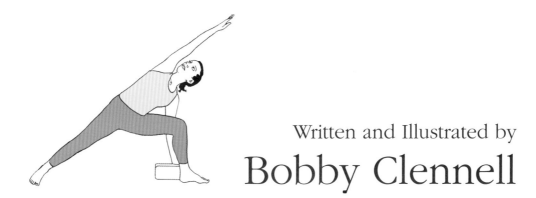

Written and Illustrated by

Bobby Clennell

Foreword by Geeta S. Iyengar, Author of *Yoga: A Gem for Women*

RODMELL PRESS • BERKELEY, CALIFORNIA • 2007

Library of Congress Cataloging-in-Publication Data

Clennell, Bobby, 1943-
   The woman's yoga book : asana and pranayama for all phases of the menstrual cycle / written and illustrated by Bobby Clennell ; foreword by Geena S. Iyengar — 1st ed.
       p. cm.
   Includes index.
   ISBN 1-930485-18-2 (pbk. : alk. paper)
   1. Yoga—Health aspects—Popular works. 2. Menstrual cycle—Popular works. 3. Menstruation disorders—Popular works. 4. Women—Health and hygiene—Popular works. I. Title.
   RA781.7.C58 2007
   613.7'046—dc22
                                        2006038298

Printed and bound in China
First Edition
ISBN-10: 1-930485-18-2
ISBN-13: 978-1-930485-18-1

17 16   3 4 5 6

Editor: Linda Cogozzo
Associate Editor: Holly Hammond
Indexer: Ty Koontz
Cover and Text Design: Gopa & Ted2, Inc.
Author Photographer: Jake Clennell
Lithographer: Union Printing Company
Text set in ITC Garamond
Distributed by Publishers Group West

For my mother, Philippa Judd

Acknowledgments

THIS BOOK is based on the work of my beloved yoga teacher, B. K. S. Iyengar, who is the source of my yoga knowledge. A heartfelt thank you to Mr. Iyengar's daughter, Geeta Iyengar, for her awe-inspiring teaching and especially for her dedicated and innovative work in the field of women's yoga.

This book could not have been written were it not for the hard work of some talented people. I would like to thank my publishers, Linda Cogozzo and Donald Moyer. Linda helped me collect and organize my thoughts, and with patience and perseverance made the writing and editing process seem painless and seamless. Thank you to Mary Talbot, who helped me find my voice in the early stages of writing, and to Lara Owen and Vivien Goldman who contributed to the preliminary editing process. I am deeply indebted to Iyengar Yoga teachers Joan White, Chris Saudek, and Lois Steinberg for their insights. Lois allowed me to spend inordinate amounts of time picking her brain. This book would not be as coherent as it is without her help.

Special thanks to my husband Lindsey, for his love and unconditional support. With his long experience as a yoga teacher and his unique abilities as a writer, he was always ready to offer a little literary fairy dust when I needed it. Lindsey and Hisayo Kushida took hundreds of photographs of me, on which I based the illustrations. A huge bouquet of red roses to each of you! Thank you also to my sons, Miles and Jake, for their love and encouragement.

For assistance with individual chapters, I acknowledge Frank Lipman, M.D., L.Ac.; Maryanne Travaglioni, L.Ac.; Harriet Beinfield, L.Ac.; and Efrem Korngold, L.Ac., O.M.D. I also thank Marcel Pick, R.N.C., M.S.N., N.P., and Leslie Boyde, M.D., for their help. Thank you to Roberta Atti for her wisdom and advice on the healing power of food.

I owe much to my friends and yoga students: Peter Simmons, Rob Gagnon, Joan Snyder, Maggie Cammer, and Diane von Furstenberg. Thank you to the many fine Iyengar Yoga teachers who helped in so many ways: Brooke Myers, Jean Marie Derrick, Yvonne Decock, Alison Pomroy, Sally Rutskey, Carrie Owerko, and Rajiv Mehta. Thank you to the late Penny Nield-Smith, Silvia Prescott, Mary Dunn, John Schumacher, Jawahar Bangera, Gabriella Giubilaro, and Stephanie Quirk.

And last but not least, a big thank you to my yoga students, who give me much more than they could ever know.

Contents

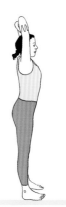

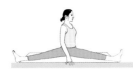

第3贴　反面 凯源-4色-WomandYoga-内页拼版.job

Foreword

By Geeta S. Iyengar

THE POPULARITY OF YOGA is increasing day by day, and it is delights my heart that many more people are embracing yoga today, as compared to the past. There was a time when many felt that yoga was meant only for recluses. However, today they understand the importance of yoga in daily life. There once was a mindset that yoga was meant exclusively for men. People realize now that this ancient art and philosophy was also a way of life for women of the Vedic period.

Yoga has a great potency to yield physical and mental health, which is essential for women. However, women should not forget its spiritual depth. The ancestral dynasty of women in yoga proves that besides physical health, they also strived for spiritual health to enrich their lives. Their endeavor did not make them turn their backs on their worldly and family responsibilities. This balance has to be struck by women of today, when the modern way of life makes them forget their womanhood.

The first stage of womanhood is menarche. In olden days, this event was celebrated as a girl's second birth; there was a naming ceremony and her horoscope (birth chart) was drawn. Thus her life was molded such that she could improve her physical, moral, mental, and spiritual health.

I grew up witnessing the importance of yoga in my life. I could sense that the practice of yoga was developing a new personality in me by bringing inner balance. As I began teaching yoga, these imprints surfaced, so I could help and educate others.

Teaching yoga in the 1960s was an adventure. Though the women were keen to learn, they had health problems. They wanted natural remedies instead of painkillers. At the time, it was not widely known that many of their problems, whether physical, psychological, or emotional, are related to menstruation and hormonal changes. I understood that link, and my method of teaching helped the women, though it took the female students a long time to adopt this view. Research today proves this link. Hence, a woman should respect her femininity and practice yoga accordingly.

Bobby Clennell rightly focuses on the practice of yoga during the different phases of menstruation, so this book is very useful for a woman from her menarche to menopause. Women will find answers to many problems they might face during that time of life. Each chapter explains the benefits of practicing the asana, while also cautioning the practitioner about what not to do and when not to do.

The journey of yoga starts with standing asanas, stabilizes one in sitting asanas, creates mobility in lateral extensions, settles one in forward extensions, brings restoration in supine asanas, refreshes one by bringing inner balance in inversions, rejuvenates the brain and nerves in backward extensions, and energizes one through pranayama. Bobby takes the reader through this entire journey. Her clear illustrations further enhance the value of the book.

I hope it will guide one and all.

Introduction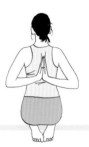

Of all the changes that have taken place throughout the last century, perhaps the most radical have been those in the lives of women. For the first time in history, many women in the West expect to take their place alongside men in the professional arena. But as women's opportunities and successes have expanded, their happiness and well-being have not always kept pace. In fact, women may be paying a price for "having it all."

Many women find that the accelerated pace of life threatens to undermine their health, erode their sense of self, and shake their spiritual center. The pressure of living up to expectations adds to the stress of a hectic schedule. This stress, along with other aspects of modern life, such as environmental pollutants and junk food, can contribute to the breakdown of the immune system and disturbances of the hormone system, putting women at risk for problems such as fibroid tumors, endometriosis, ovarian cysts, and menstrual irregularities.

Without a doubt, the pattern of menstruation has been altered by postindustrial life. Because today's woman starts her period earlier and has fewer babies, she can have between 350 and 400 menstrual periods throughout her lifetime, as opposed to the 100 periods that most women experienced two hundred years ago. At one time, pregnancy and lactation provided respite from the monthly period, but women now have far fewer children than their foremothers, and many do not have children at all. This change, plus the demands that women face in the modern world, may be forcing the female reproductive system to adapt in unhealthy ways. Whether we have children or not, women are focused on "keeping up." Listening to internal needs falls low on the list of priorities, and inevitably many women adopt unhealthy lifestyles, hardly noticing what is happening in our bodies.

Some women ignore the very thing that makes us different from men: cyclical hormonal rhythms. And for all of our advances in social equality, attitudes toward menstruation are only slightly more enlightened than in the past. The once prevailing notion that a menstruating woman was unclean has been replaced by an attitude of neglect, both by society and by women themselves. On one hand, women may have an increased number of menstrual periods; on the other hand, we are no longer encouraged to think of menstruation as a significant or spiritual event. There is virtually no remaining tradition in Western culture that acknowledges the power and mystery of the menstrual cycle. Many women's magazines, the bellwethers of contemporary female culture, do not encourage us to rest or meditate at this time.

1

Instead, we are told to go to the gym, highlight our hair, and get over it.

How can we as women rediscover our unique creative power and live holistically without compromising our recently won and crucially important place in society? In *The Woman's Yoga Book*, I do not ask you to return to the repressive attitudes of the prefeminist era, or to abandon your independence for a life of continual pregnancy and childbirth. I suggest instead that feminism take into consideration the biological reality of womanhood. My intention is to offer all women—whether they have children or not, whether they have careers or not—the teachings of a wise, age-old system of healing that is ours for the taking: yoga.

My Personal Journey

I discovered yoga while living in London. It was 1973, and I had two young sons, Miles and Jake. Propelled by a friend's enthusiastic recommendations, my husband, Lindsey, and I took our first yoga class. It was with Penny Nield-Smith, in a community center in Covent Garden. We were hooked immediately. It was only later that we learned that this kind of yoga was called Iyengar Yoga, after B. K. S. Iyengar, author of *Light on Yoga*. In 1975 I made my first journey to India to study with Iyengar himself, his daughter Geeta S. Iyengar, author of *Yoga: A Gem for Women*, and his son, Prashant Iyengar. My life was changed by this experience. In particular, I was absolutely enthralled by Geeta Iyengar's insights and wisdom about women and yoga. I began teaching in 1976, when Penny handed over the weekly Covent Garden class to me.

As a young mother juggling the demands of family and work in a changing and sometimes overwhelming world, yoga gave me the means to achieve physical strength, emotional stability, confidence, and courage. When my period came around each month, I made sure that there was time to practice a calming restorative sequence, regardless of the other demands on me.

This sequence, which was specific to menstruation, took approximately an hour and a half. I practiced it every day of my period. Soon I discovered that if in addition to this I remained as still and as quiet as possible after work on the days of the heaviest bleeding, then things went better for me throughout the rest of the month. A few years earlier a vegetarian diet and the macrobiotic movement had awakened me from the stodginess of traditional English cooking and the sterility of frozen fish fingers! My early cooking experiments set the groundwork for my developing interest in how everything that I did influenced my body–mind. My monthly yoga ritual not only helped me overcome menstrual discomfort but also (along with the rest of my practice) helped to broaden my perspective on my place in the world beyond my day-to-day concerns.

Throughout the years, I have kept up with my yoga practice, refining it to meet my needs. I have returned to India, time and again, to study with the Iyengars. I have found myself increasingly focused on women's issues in yoga. Thousands of women practice yoga today, often with the knowledge that keeping their bodies supple and free of tension is a good antidote to stiffness and the aging effects of stress. But yoga is not only positive for flexibility and relaxation; it is also a powerful healing tool. Many of the asana (yoga poses) and pranayama (breathing practices) act as tonics and regulators for a woman's reproductive system. As a yoga teacher, I have observed how women's lives have been transformed as a result of practicing yoga with attention to their cycles.

The cyclic nature of women's physiology binds

us inextricably to the natural world, and when this bond is weakened, humankind as a whole suffers. A yoga practice that includes attention to the rhythmic patterns of our female energy can strengthen our connection to the cycles of nature and can, in a small way, help to restore balance to the planet. With intelligent yoga practice, a woman becomes an active participant in her own health care. By reclaiming the power to heal ourselves, we also reclaim the power to heal others.

About This Book

The Woman's Yoga Book is a comprehensive approach to practicing yoga to balance, regulate, and honor your menstrual cycle, whether you are new to yoga or a continuing student. Chapter 1 presents an overview of the history of menstrual beliefs and practices, examining how modern concepts developed and how ancient traditions from profeminine cultures can help us regain a healthy perspective on this most essential of body rhythms. Chapter 2 covers the basic physiology of menstruation and discusses the relationship between physiological events and emotional changes during the month.

Chapter 3 explains how Iyengar Yoga is particularly useful for women and which asana and pranayama work best at what stage of the monthly cycle. Chapter 4 explores the fundamentals of setting up a regular yoga practice. Chapters 5 through 11 give step-by-step instructions in asana and pranayama and how women should practice them. Chapters 12 through 14 describe practice sequences to keep your menstrual cycle healthy and keep you attuned to your nature as a woman.

Finally, chapters 15 through 23 present sequences that are specifically designed for different menstrual problems, ranging from irritability to excessive menstrual flow. You can refer back to chapters 5 through 11 at any time, for the detailed instructions on any the poses presented in these sequences. At the back of the book is a comprehensive list of resources to aid your yoga practice.

I invite you to use *The Woman's Yoga Book* to help you practice yoga in ways that meet your needs and to empower you with the means to balance your menstrual cycle throughout the month. I wish you much joy and comfort from your yoga practice.

Ancient Teachings and Modern Concepts

THE WOMAN'S YOGA BOOK focuses on using yoga to balance and regulate the reproductive cycle throughout the month. Before we look at how to do that, let's examine how menstruation has been viewed at different times in history and by different cultures. By exploring a variety of belief systems and attitudes, including current Western thinking, we can begin to heal our bodies and psyches from centuries of mistrust of the female body.

The Cultures of Menstruation

Menstruation has not always been considered either a curse to be feared and reviled or a biological necessity to be ignored. In profeminine cultures, menstruation was seen as a precious time for seeking inner knowledge and self-renewal. In many cultures, the blood itself was considered to have immense power, especially the first blood that signals a girl's transition to womanhood. Menstrual blood was deemed magical and guaranteed fertility. Penelope Shuttle and Peter Redgrove, in their groundbreaking book on menstruation *The Wise Wound: Menstruation and Everywoman,* claim that the first shamans, prophets, and priests were women, most likely because they were perceived as powerful as a consequence of menstruation. Archeological evi-

dence strongly suggests that menstrual blood was once revered as the source of life. Among the Navaho, for instance, when a girl first began to bleed, the whole tribe celebrated this reassurance that life would go on.

Throughout history, menstruating women have been variously isolated, feared, avoided, envied, insulted, and in some cases worshipped. But whether or not a society's attitude was negative or positive, it reflected an appreciation of women's potency. Only recently has menstruation been almost completely ignored, both by women themselves and by the surrounding culture.

In Orthodox Judaism, menstruating women are admonished to refrain from touching the Torah, or Holy Scriptures. Interpretations of this vary: either a woman's power is so great during menstruation that she might harm sacred objects, or she is unclean and might contaminate them. Whatever the reason, she is kept away from the holy books, the sources of spiritual power.

In contrast, other cultures have seen the menstruating woman as particularly in harmony with the realm of spirit. In Australian aboriginal culture, women are considered sacred for the duration of their periods. According to Robert Lawler, author of *Voices of the First Day: Awakening in the Aboriginal Dreamtime,* menstrual blood is considered so powerful that women are not allowed to conceal that they are menstruating..

In many cultures, women are taught to avoid sexual intercourse during menstruation. Orthodox Jewish couples abide by laws of *niddah,* or "family purity." During a wife's period and for seven days afterward, couples must abstain from sexual contact, sleep in separate beds, and express affection in nonphysical ways. An Orthodox Jewish woman then undergoes a ritual cleansing, in which she immerses herself for at least thirty minutes in the *mikveh,* or "collection of water," which is like a miniature indoor swimming pool. Likewise, in some Muslim cultures, women are required to suspend sexual intercourse during menstruation. Similar to the Jewish custom of ritual bathing, they fully immerse and wash themselves in water, known as *ghul,* once the bleeding has stopped.

Chinese women are also taught to avoid sexual intercourse during menses. In *Traditional Chinese Medicine,* Nan Lu, O.M.D., notes that because women are energetically more vulnerable during their periods, having sex at this time might cause a menstrual cycle disorder, such as painful periods, cramping, and longer periods. He points out that infection is more readily transferable between partners during menstruation.

In other cultures, it is believed that women emit a different energy during menstruation. Some Native American tribes believed that menstruating women interfered with the energy of men and prevented them from fighting well during battle. In Spain and France, this energy was thought to contaminate food. For example, menstruating women could not make mayonnaise because it was thought that the eggs would not bind.

In India, this energy is also thought to contaminate food. But Geeta Iyengar, who is trained in ayurveda, India's traditional system of health and healing, has a less insulting take on the bad-

energy theory. She describes menstrual energy as heat that is thrown out of the body. (We will work with this principle later in the book.)

In addition, Geeta explains that in India women are indeed kept away from the main hub of family life and are excused from cooking during menses. At times and in climates where infectious disease is prevalent, this separation is intended to protect women, because their immune systems are somewhat weakened during menstruation. The Indian system offers another advantage: rest at a time when a woman's energy is at its lowest ebb.

A female Muslim yoga student whom I met in New York told me that outsiders interpret traditional practices of this kind as reflections of the oppression of women. In fact, she observed, Muslim women are grateful for the opportunity to rest. As India becomes more Westernized, however, these ancient traditions are in danger of disappearing.

In other Indian traditions, menstruation is considered a sacred event. In Tantra, a woman embodies different forms of the goddess, depending on her place in her monthly cycle. During menstruation itself, she is seen as beyond the world and its responsibilities and therefore freed from household duties. It is during this time that she serves as a link between this world and the next.

Is Menstruation Obsolete?

According to biologist Beverly Strassmann, who teaches at the University of Michigan at Ann Arbor, the once-monthly period is a relatively new phenomenon in the history of menstruation. Strassmann studied the Dogon women in Mali, Africa, for two and a half years. She found that, on average, the Dogon woman has her first period at age sixteen and gives birth eight or nine times. She spends so much time either pregnant or breastfeeding that she averages only slightly more than one period a year. All told, Dogon women menstruate about 100 times in their lives. Strassmann believes that the basic pattern of late menarche, many pregnancies, and long, menstrual-free stretches caused by intensive breastfeeding was virtually universal until the demographic transition from high to low fertility that occurred a hundred years ago. By contrast, Western woman menstruate somewhere between 350 and 400 times.

Meanwhile, according to scholar Stephen T. Chang, author of *The Tao of Sexology,* women of the ancient courts of China used Taoist practices, which included breathing techniques and massage, to suspend their periods indefinitely as a way to remain young and beautiful. According to Taoist belief, while men lose their energy through ejaculation, women lose most of their energy through menstruation. In other words, Chang claims that the shedding of the ovaries causes a woman to age.

In some quarters, Western allopathic medicine may be coming closer to the Taoist belief that continual, unabated menstrual bleeding is harmful for the body. In his controversial book *Is Menstruation Obsolete?*, gynecologist Elsimar M. Coutinho suggests that menstruation is an unhealthy and unnecessary process. He advocates suppressing ovulation and therefore monthly bleeding artificially with specially formulated hormones, similar to the birth control pill. (Before we allow this idea to gain momentum, we should remember other instances in which we have allowed ourselves to be used as human laboratories, such as to test the birth control pill and hormone replacement therapy.)

In ayurveda, menstruation is considered to be a regulating process that corrects any imbalances that may have occurred in the preceding month. Men's bodies do not have such a mechanism. Ayurvedic physician, scholar, and author Robert Svoboda suggests that this regulating mechanism, via menstruation, may be one reason why women live longer than men. While the ayurvedic view sees a woman's monthly period as a healthy mechanism, it also links menstruation with certain health risks. In *Ayurveda for Women: A Guide to Vitality and Health,* Svoboda observes that because women have more periods now than in previous times, they are more vulnerable to the accompanying hormonal shifts, each of which strongly affects the tissues of their ovaries, uterus, and breasts. These hormonal swings are opportunities for imbalances to occur or for existing imbalances to be exacerbated. If this is true, all the more reason for a woman to preserve her menstrual balance and take care of herself throughout the month.

Once a girl's cycle becomes regular, she can expect to menstruate approximately once a month unless she becomes pregnant. This makes for a lot of periods in one lifetime. Other than to provide a suitable environment for a new life, what could menstruation be for? There is no consensus on why women bleed, although theories about the matter abound. I embrace the views of ayurveda and Western medicine that menstruation is a cleansing process. But it may help us to place menstruation in perspective to look at a few other attitudes on women's reproductive cycles.

In *Woman: An Intimate Geography,* author Natalie Angier discusses Margie Profet, an evolutionary biologist at the University of Washington, who is the first woman scientist to ask the question, Why do women menstruate? Profet puts forth the provocative theory that menstruation is a defense mechanism and an extension of the body's immune system. She suggests that monthly bleeding flushes out harmful microbes that might enter a woman's body on the backs of sperm during intercourse. The response to Profet's theory from gynecologists and other specialists in the field has been overwhelmingly negative. Far from being a protective mechanism, they argue, women are more at risk for bacterial infections during the bleeding phase of menstruation. Profet's most valuable contribution may have been to take the lid off a subject that had not only been neglected by the (mostly male) scientific community but that was also largely taboo.

Angier also writes about Beverly Strassmann, a biologist at the University of Michigan at Ann Arbor, who offers another explanation on why women bleed. Although it is not yet fully understood how the human being developed such a large brain relative to other mammalian species, there does appear to be a correlation between brain capacity and the mother's placenta. The brain and complex nervous system of human beings evolved, at least in part, due to the extraordinarily abundant nourishment supplied by the mother via the placenta to the baby growing inside her. Menstrual blood flow, Strassmann argues, is part of the same process that provides blood to the growing fetus. She further points out that animals with less brain function have less nourishing placenta and bleed either not at all or very little when they are in season.

Strassmann has come up with another interesting observation. She notes that maintaining the endometrial lining during the second half of the ovarian cycle takes substantial metabolic energy. If pregnancy does not take place, it makes energetic sense for the endometrium to be sloughed off and to regenerate itself, rather than to maintain unneeded tissue. Such energy conservation is common among vertebrates: male rhesus monkeys' testes shrink during their nonbreeding season, Burmese pythons' guts shrink when they are not digesting, and the metabolisms of hibernating animals are put on hold.

From this brief overview, we can see that menstruation and menstrual blood have elicited all kinds of reactions throughout history, and that even today science struggles to understand the mysteries of the menstrual cycle. (See resources for further reading on the subject.)

There is still so much we don't know about women's hormonal rhythms, about what affects our cycles, and about how we can best live in harmony with our bodies. What we do know is that each of us holds innate knowledge about our own rhythms, and that any practice that encourages greater self-awareness and body-mind interconnectedness can help us tune in to our inner wisdom more readily. I do not suggest that we overcome biology but that, through the practice of yoga, we learn to work with it.

2

From Menarche to Menopause: Cycles of a Woman's Life

URING HER LIFETIME, a woman undergoes a series of developmental stages that bring about profound physiological and psychological transformations. As we saw in chapter 1, each of these stages has been perceived differently by women and their communities throughout history and across cultures. Feminine rites of passage, such as a girl's first period, are cause for celebration in some societies and a source of ritual banishment in others. But whatever the prevailing belief system of traditional societies, a woman's body and its cycles have always had deep resonance for her and for the people around her.

Menarche

The onset of menstruation is called *menarche,* from the Greek for month (*men*) and beginning (*arkhe).* Two hundred years ago the average age of menarche was seventeen. Now most girls start their periods earlier, at around twelve or thirteen years of age, with some beginning as early as ten. This is partly due to modern nutrition: our diets are richer in the fats and proteins needed to bring a girl to the critical weight—approximately 110 pounds—that she must attain for menstruation to begin. Girls who are heavier tend to menstruate earlier than girls who weigh less. In *Ayurveda for Women: A Guide to Vitality and Health,* Robert Svoboda cites other factors that may speed up the normal course of events, such as light and the hormones that are added to the diets of farm-raised animals, which we in turn consume. Both strong sunlight and artificial light influence brain and body chemistry. Girls in Mediterranean countries, where the light level is high all year round, used to reach maturity at an earlier age than girls in regions that receive less sun. Now, living under electric lights may hasten the onset of menarche for girls all over the world.

For a young girl entering puberty, a few years may pass before ovulation occurs on a regular basis. In the first years that a girl menstruates, hormone levels often fluctuate considerably before settling down. It is normal for a young woman to have an irregular cycle in the early stages of her puberty.

The hormonal upheavals that accompany puberty also subject many girls to disrupted sleeping patterns, particularly in the week preceding menstruation. Teenage girls sometimes need to sleep a lot, unlike menopausal women, who may have problems sleeping at all. Mood and behavioral changes may also accompany the first few years of menstruation. These changes vary widely

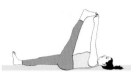

from girl to girl, just as women's experience of menopause is similarly individual. However, as pointed out by Penelope Shuttle and Peter Redgrove in *The Wise Wound: The Myths, Realities, and Meanings of Menstruation,* one characteristic is shared by all pubescent girls: increased daydreaming.

This is a fascinating finding, especially when one considers that what in the West is interpreted as moodiness or absentmindedness is seen as heightened awareness in other cultures. Shuttle and Redgrove note that in one Mojave Indian tradition a girl in her "moon time" was instructed to remember the details of her dreams and recount them to her elders. It was from these dreams that her future life was predicted.

What the Mojave and other tribal societies knew is that menarche is a woman's initiation into adulthood. It is a natural and embodied event, stimulated by hormone changes that predispose her to inner visions. The young men of African and Native American tribal societies are taken on vision quests in order to get this same quality of information.

The Menstrual Cycle: Time and Tide

A woman's monthly cycle mirrors the cyclical nature of the universe and is of the same duration as the moon's cycle—approximately 29.5 days. Various studies made in the early 1900s found that a significant number of menstrual cycles started at the full moon or the new moon, although the interval between periods can vary considerably among women. Depending on their age, energetic tendencies, and lifestyle, the interval can range from 20 to 40 days.

The earth's waters, of which women's menstrual fluids are a part, move in rhythms. We are influenced by the earth, the moon, and the sun, and also by the women around us. Women who spend prolonged periods of time together often find that their menstrual cycles begin to synchronize.

The study that first alerted the scientific community to the notion that pheromones (airborne chemicals) can influence the timing of women's menstrual cycles was conducted in 1974 by biologist Martha McClintock at the University of Chicago. In a later experiment, McClintock again demonstrated that pheromones can send out strong messages. By taking swabs from the armpits of women at different points of their ovulatory cycle and applying them to the upper lips of other women, ovulation could be hastened or slowed in the recipient.

Subsequent tests showed however that, as the months passed, some cohabiting women became distinctly "less harmonized." Natalie Angier, author of *Woman: An Intimate Geography,* who interviewed McClintock, observes that many factors come into play in the unconscious signals women send to each other.

In *Ayurveda: Secrets of Healing,* Maya Tiwari notes that when the menstrual cycle has not been affected by the use of contraceptive pills, harmful foods, and other disruptive activities, it remains in harmony with the cycles of the moon. Many ancient tribal cultures observed that women ovulated on the full moon and menstruated on the new moon.

In *Blood Magic: The Anthropology of Menstruation,* anthropologist Thomas Buckley cites a Yurok woman who reported that in old-time village life women from the same household menstruated at the same time, which was thought to be dictated by the moon. If a woman found that her menstrual cycle was out of sync with the other women and therefore with the moon, she would sit in the moonlight and ask the moon to balance her. This is interesting in view of the finding that light stimulates ovulation, particularly when a woman is exposed to it while sleeping.

Lara Owen, author of *Honoring Menstruation: A Time of Self–Renewal,* points out that in our postindustrial society artificial light may have confused the ovulation cycle. Moonlight is only one of the many nocturnal light sources we are now exposed to, which may be why our periods no longer coincide with the cycles of the moon.

Whereas Western-trained physicians tend not to be concerned if women's cycles are irregular, doctors of Chinese medicine and ayurveda watch for subtle signs of imbalance, because they know that that these can indicate a potential for future illness. Stress, inadequate diet, overvigorous exercise, light deprivation, and travel can all disrupt menstrual rhythms.

The Physiology of the Menstrual Cycle

The menstrual cycle is governed by interactions between the hypothalamus gland (located deep in the brain), the pituitary gland (located at the base of the brain, level with the eyes), and the two almond-shaped ovaries attached to the uterus (located in the lower abdomen). Together these glands form a loop of coordinated hormonal messages, upon which the health and stability of the menstrual cycle depends.

The first day of bleeding is considered the first day of the cycle. A period usually lasts from three to five days, and the flow of blood varies in intensity. For some women, the flow is heaviest at the beginning of menstruation, while for others it is heaviest in the middle or toward the end. Healthy menstrual blood is deep carmine in color. The volume of blood expelled on average is less than a quarter of a cup, or six tablespoons, with each period. (Put another way, we discard forty quarts of blood and fluid over a lifetime of menses!) Accompanying hormonal changes influence the way we feel. Some women experience a release of tension with the onset of menstruation, as estrogen levels drop. This release however is not generally accompanied by a boost in energy. Around the start of menstruation, as both progesterone and estrogen levels are at their lowest, a woman may be more susceptible than usual to infections and viruses. She may also feel tired or experience a lack of focus; she may not feel like doing anything. The period is finished when the red blood flow tapers off and combines with the normal cervical and vaginal secretions, first turning to brown and then disappearing completely.

In my early days of studying with Geeta Iyengar, I was most intrigued by her observance of a postmenstrual phase. Geeta teaches that the chemical changes that take place in the body following menstruation can signal mood swings not unlike postnatal euphoria. This is in no way debilitating or dramatic; in fact, it is very subtle. When we practice yoga, we become better able to observe the various fluctuations in our energy throughout the month. During the four days following menstruation, when estrogen levels begin to surge, we should select asana that help us maintain emotional stability and hormonal balance. (See chapter 13.)

In addition, Geeta points out that following menstruation, the uterus, which has just been working hard, is in recovery mode and needs to relax. Yurok women, along with women from other tribal societies and cultures, including orthodox Jewish women, also observe the postmenstrual phase. Not only do they separate from

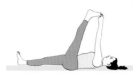

men during the active bleeding phase of menstruation but also for the four or five days following, making it ten days in all.

During the first half of the cycle, from menstruation until ovulation, estrogen levels are rising, and follicle-stimulating hormone (FSH) is directing the ovarian follicles to grow an egg large enough to be ovulated, to be erupted from the ovarian wall. This is an expansive time, during which estrogen dominates and strongly influences a woman's system. Estrogen has a rejuvenating effect: it conditions the hair, makes the skin bloom, and lifts the mood. You feel optimistic, as if you can tackle anything.

Estrogen causes the lining of the uterus to thicken, as it prepares to house a possibly fertilized egg. Around twelve to sixteen days into the cycle, estrogen levels rise again, this time dramatically, and the pituitary gland secretes a sudden surge of luteinizing hormone (LH). The egg erupts from the wall of the ovary, and ovulation takes place, usually unnoticed, over the next forty-eight hours. (Some women experience a twinge in the area of the ovaries, and others experience spotting or a heightened sense of sight or smell.) When ovulation takes place, many women experience an increased sex drive, which is nature's way of making pregnancy more likely. For some women, the estrogen surge can trigger a migraine headache.

The egg is then funneled into one of the waiting fallopian tubes and is wafted down into the warmth and protection of the uterus. Fluctuations in the consistency of cervical mucus secretions throughout the month provide clues as to whether or not ovulation has taken place. A plug of thick mucus expelled from the cervix can be the first sign of imminent ovulation. Around the time of ovulation, mucus production increases

and takes on the consistency of raw egg white—expansive, stretchy, and clear. Following ovulation, secretions become pastier and thicker.

Within hours of ovulation, hormone levels make another dramatic shift: the empty follicle begins to excrete progesterone, which now dominates the hormone balance. Progesterone, which reaches its peak around days nineteen to twenty-one, causes the secretion of a special sugar that makes the uterus soft and spongy, helping to prepare it for pregnancy.

The second half of the cycle can be a contemplative, reflective phase for a woman, or it can be very uncomfortable. Premenstrual syndrome (PMS) affects increasing numbers of women. Its occurrence coincides with urbanization and the accelerated pace of life, and with the accompanying changes in diet and lifestyle. PMS can also occur when the menstrual cycle is not honored. Monica Sjoo and Barbara Mor, in their inspiring book *The Great Cosmic Mother: Rediscovering the Religion of the Earth*, propose that premenstrual tension is caused by ignoring an increased need to dream and meditate.

In *Once a Month: Understanding and Treating P.M.S.,* Katherine Dalton defines PMS as the occurrence of symptoms before menstruation that are completely absent after menstruation. Dalton notes that there are some 150 different recorded symptoms. Other researchers have recorded more than 200 symptoms of PMS, but women who suffer from it usually experience only 2 or 3 of them at any given time.

Among the most common premenstrual symptoms are mood swings, irritability, inability to concentrate, migraine headaches, sore and swollen breasts, and food cravings. Some women experience heightened awareness of self during this phase, and it can be a time of great insight and vision. It really depends on how things are going in a woman's life. Feelings that may have been bubbling under the surface throughout the month may boil over in the days leading up to menstruation. Frustrations, unexpressed anger, and unfulfilled dreams become more difficult to ignore. During perimenopause, the years leading up to the full cessation of periods, PMS may become even more intense, due to the increased fluctuation of hormones and erratic menstrual cycles.

At the end of the cycle, two to three days prior to menstruation, if fertilization has not occurred, the ovaries cease to secrete hormones. Without hormones to support its growth, the lining of the uterus deteriorates and shrinks. It is then sloughed off and, together with blood, other secretions, and the unfertilized egg, it is discharged through the cervix and flows out through the vagina. Menstruation has begun, and the cycle starts anew.

Menopause

Menopause is the natural termination of the menstrual cycle and a woman's reproductive years. Although 10 percent of women in the United States begin menopause before age forty, it usually occurs around fifty-one years of age. The complete transition lasts approximately six to thirteen years. This includes the postmenopausal phase, when women often experience symptoms that reflect a settling down of hormonal shifts.

During menopause, the menstrual cycle undergoes radical changes. Women have a limited number of eggs stored in the ovaries and, as they reach their forties, they occasionally have cycles where ovulation doesn't occur. Consequently, as estrogen and progesterone levels become more erratic, so do their periods. One to three years before the onset of the permanent cessation of menses, women often miss one or more periods. They may find that when menstruation does occur, it is more frequent. Women in perimenopause may experience low-estrogen months, when hot flashes are experienced, along with a light or scanty period. This may be followed by a high-estrogen month, when the hot flashes disappear and when they experience breast pain and heavy bleeding.

Postmenopausal women are often much more attuned to their internal power and intuitive feelings than they were earlier in life. No longer at the mercy of constantly cycling hormones, they often find they have extra energy to direct to the spiritual, creative, and social areas of their lives. As women continue to raise awareness about the role of older women in society, it becomes more obvious than ever that we need the contribution of these experienced and mature women in all areas of our global culture.

3
How Yoga Can Help Women

YOGA, as we know it today, dates from approximately 2500 B.C.E. It is derived from a system of psychology, medicine, and cosmic law that has its roots in the Indus Valley civilization of India. The word *yoga,* translated from the Sanskrit, literally means "union." Its fundamental purpose is to unite the mind with the body and to reintegrate individual consciousness with universal consciousness. Experiencing this union and reintegration can occur when asana and pranayama are practiced regularly.

As such, yoga has a healing effect on the body, mind, and spirit. Indeed, yoga is holistic healing in the most profound sense: it stimulates the body's innate ability to heal itself. Different asana and pranayama act on the body in different ways, affecting not only the muscles and joints but also the respiratory, digestive, circulatory, nervous, immune, endocrine, and reproductive systems. It balances the subtle energies of mind and body, calms and steadies the nerves, and dramatically reduces physical tension. When we practice yoga, we are better able to put our problems into perspective. We can't pretend they don't exist; we still have to deal with them. But with the physical, mental, and emotional flexibility that yoga gives us, we can move more easily, bend and flow with the stresses of life.

The Iyengars

I practice and teach yoga in the tradition of B. K. S. Iyengar, an internationally renowned yoga master who has taught for over sixty years. His Ramamani Iyengar Memorial Yoga Institute, in Pune, India, has produced a worldwide network of teachers and training centers that continues to grow steadily. Today there are more than 2,000 certified Iyengar teachers around the globe.

Mr. Iyengar is the author of several highly acclaimed books, including the yoga classic *Light on Yoga.* Throughout the years, he has developed his method of yoga into the precise science that it is today. He is especially sought-after for his genius in understanding health problems and for adapting asana and pranayama for therapeutic use.

In the 1930s, in a culture where women had few rights, Mr. Iyengar began teaching yoga to women. At that time Indian women were discouraged from practicing yoga on the grounds that it might make them less feminine. They were also hesitant to learn yoga from male teachers, but since he was then a young boy, his guru assigned him to teach the women. It was against much opposition that he endeavored to find the correct practices for women.

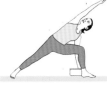

In 1975, when I first traveled to Pune to study with Mr. Iyengar, I was struck by the inclusiveness of his classes. As an English woman, I was used to the boys-club atmosphere of my homeland. This, along with my somewhat introverted personality, resulted in my tendency to stand on the sidelines. Alas, Mr. Iyengar would have none of it! His teaching style and his expectations of students is legendary. Regardless of one's creed, gender, or age, there is no hiding from him. He still demands that his students be fully present and fully engaged when he is teaching.

Mr. Iyengar's daughter Geeta has followed in her father's footsteps and is a dynamic exponent of his teaching. She has made the women's aspect of her father's work her specialty. I learned the basics of my menstrual practice from her, and through it I healed my own menstrual problems. During my twenty-three-year teaching career, thanks to Mr. Iyengar's and Geeta's dedication to yoga, I have also been able to help many students with chronic menstrual cramps, absence of menstruation, heavy menstrual flow, and other difficulties.

Why Yoga Is Especially Good for Women

We all know that we need some form of exercise to stay healthy. A study led by Anne McTiernan, principal investigator and director of the Fred Hutchinson Cancer Research Center in Seattle, Washington, found that exercise lowers levels of blood estrogen in postmenopausal women. In a similar study, Leslie Bernstein, professor of preventive medicine at the University of Southern California School of Medicine, found that women in the under-forty age group who exercised for at least four hours each week during their reproductive years were 50 percent less likely to develop breast cancer than women who didn't

exercise. Bernstein also discovered that estrogen depletion has a less happy outcome when it occurs in young girls going through puberty. Even moderate amounts of activity can increase the length of menstrual cycles and reduce the number of times a girl ovulates.

Menstrual irregularity is fairly common among young women who exercise to excess. Young women athletes often experience disturbance in their menstrual cycles, with skipped periods and sometimes no periods at all. If periods stop altogether (a condition known as amenorrhea), women can lose so much calcium from their bones that they can develop osteoporosis while they are still young. Some of my students have traced their irregularity to a time when they were working out rigorously on a regular basis.

It is clear that hormone levels are both affected by exercise and influence the body's reaction to it. An ongoing study conducted by Edward M. Wojtys, an orthopedic surgeon at the University of Michigan at Ann Arbor, shows that during ovulation (when estrogen production is high) women have about three times the average number of knee injuries than during other times of the month, and are up to eight times more likely to sustain knee injuries than men. As yet, no firm conclusions have been drawn from this study, but it does point to a link between hormone fluctuations and injuries.

There is no denying that exercise is beneficial, and there is no denying that it has its drawbacks. For example, while aerobic exercise stimulates cardiovascular activity and reduces high estrogen levels, it wears out the joints. Running, for instance, places a tremendous stress on the lower extremities, and approximately 60 percent of the 30 million Americans who run will experience an injury that may limit their activities.

Many of the exercise choices that women make

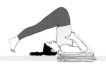

are done in the spirit of competition. We may feel that we have to keep our bodies thin, hard, and muscular, like men's bodies. This is understandable, because women now compete with men (and each other) in the workplace. But many exercise regimes deplete women, or are inadequate for women, or both. For example, I have seen extensive damage done to the female reproductive system by weightlifting. By the time she gets to menopause, a woman weightlifter's body is hard and brittle. And the menopausal transition itself can be severely hampered by the hormone system having been ignored for so long.

Yoga is an ideal form of exercise for women because it combines cardiovascular training, muscle strengthening, and weight-bearing activity, but it does not compromise the organs, hormone system, or joints. In fact, it keeps them healthy, provided that the balance between rigor and relaxation is met. A yoga practice that is dull and without vitality will not have a positive effect on the body's systems. At the other extreme, an overzealous and aggressive yoga practice can strain the body just as much as working out on machines in the gym.

As women, we need to be aware of the cyclic nature of our physiology. We must listen carefully to our bodies and use asana and pranayama that will help at a particular time in our cycle. Practices that are suitable at midcycle, for example, are inappropriate during menstruation. And although yoga is particularly suited to the female body, which is more supple and softer than a man's, women should avoid overstretching. For instance, a woman who understands how to align her pelvic bones and stretch up through her torso and chest during yoga practice will find that low back pain, which can be one of the first indications that a woman's exercise regime is straining her internal organs, becomes a thing of the past.

In summary, a regular, well-considered yoga practice, one that takes into account the cyclic nature of a woman's body, will provide major health benefits. It will support a woman throughout all the phases of her life. It will give her the tools to overcome physical limitations, establish emotional and mental stability, and stay true to her feminine nature.

An Overview: Practicing the Right Pose at the Right Time

As women we witness a constant dance of creation and renewal played out in our bodies. Thus it is important to take a mindful and sensitive approach to the practice of yoga. Different poses produce different responses within the system. You can nurture a state of vibrant good health by doing the right poses at the right time of your cycle. This will influence your short-term and long-term reproductive health, supporting fertility and healthy menstruation and a smooth transition into menopause. Notice how you feel before and after a session of yoga and before and after each pose, as well as how your body responds to the various poses at different stages of the month. This section gives an overview of how to practice, including what to avoid and what to focus on during each phase of the menstrual cycle.

During the Menstrual Period

During the active bleeding phase of the cycle, use your yoga practice to align your body with the frequency of the earth, to gather energy, and to rest. This is the most sensitive part of the cycle, so avoid strenuous activities, like hiking, dancing, and heavy housework. (This last activity hasn't changed much with the advent of feminism:

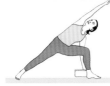

today women who work outside the home still do around 70 percent of household chores, according to author Judith Warner. We've got to stay on it, ladies. During your period, at least, delegate!) Similarly postpone energetic or demanding yoga poses, and do not turn yourself upside down.

STANDING POSES AND VINYASA FLOWING SEQUENCES. Avoid standing poses, particularly during the heavy phase of your period. A certain amount of heat is discharged from the body during menstruation, and these poses generate heat. This disturbs rather than enhances the process of elimination. Additionally the uterus should not be put through any kind of stress during menstruation. Since there is a tendency for women to tighten the lower abdomen (and so the uterus) while practicing standing poses, they are best avoided.

There are a few exceptions. Practice supported variations of Utthita Trikonasana and Ardha Chandrasana to relieve low back pain and reduce cramping, excessive bleeding, and bloating. The standing forward extensions, such as Uttanasana with Head Support, Adho Mukha Svanasana with Head Support, and Prasarita Padottanasana with Head on Block help relieve low back pain and reduce high blood pressure.

Low hormone levels during menses mean that energy should be conserved, so avoid a practice that involves jumping, such as Surya Namaskara.

SITTING POSES AND TWISTS. Sitting poses, when combined with side-bending poses like Parsva Adho Mukha Swastikasana, can reduce swelling and stiffness in the joints. They also can provide relief from low back pain, menstrual cramps, and migraine headaches. To minimize effort and avoid strain, practice them with support during this time.

During menstruation avoid deep abdominal twists, because they can pressurize the lower abdominal organs (which includes the ovaries, uterus, and vagina) and may cause flooding or clotting of menstrual blood. In gentle twists, such as Bharadvajasana II, Parsva Virasana, and Parsva Swastikasana, there is minimal disturbance to the abdominal organs. You can practice them during menstruation, as long as your flow is not heavy. They may provide a welcome relief from low back pain.

SEATED FORWARD BENDS. These poses are highly recommended for practice during menstruation. They quiet the brain and reduce headaches, backache, and fatigue. Some seated forward bends, like Janu Sirsasana with Legs Apart, can also reduce heavy bleeding.

RECLINING POSES. These asana reduce pelvic soreness and abdominal cramps, relax the nerves, and counteract fatigue. However, reclining poses that require strong abdominal work, such as Supta Padangustasana III, as well as reclining leg lifts in which the abdomen is pumped up and down, compress and irritate the internal organs and may cause the menstrual flow to become heavy. (Also avoid "crunches," the exercises often done to firm and tone the abdominal muscles. If you are doing Pilates, suspend it during menstruation, because it also involves abdominal work.)

INVERSIONS. These are the poses in which your head is lower than your torso, hips, and legs. They are contraindicated while you are bleeding. According to ayurveda, *mala,* which means "waste" (urine, feces, phlegm, mucus, and menstrual blood), has to be thrown out of the body in order to avoid disease. As such a woman's body is designed to allow the menstrual discharge to

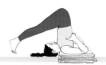

flow unrestricted. If the body is turned upside down, this process is disturbed and may force the menstrual flow to back up into the abdominal cavity and up through the fallopian tubes, causing the uterus to perform an adapted function instead of its normal function. This may contribute to endometriosis or other problems, such as cramping or insufficient or excessive menstrual flow. Since the menstrual process is one of discharge, it is a commonsense precaution to avoid these poses. Do not practice any inversions until the menstrual flow has stopped completely.

BACK BENDS. Women generally have less energy during menstruation. Back bends are stimulating poses and, when practiced during menstruation, they overtax the system at a time when women most need rest. They also can interfere with natural rhythms and in the long term can adversely affect fertility. However, one supported backbend, Viparita Dandasana II with Head and Feet Supported, is beneficial, provided you keep the reproductive organs soft and in their proper alignment within the pelvis. Practice it during menses to maintain hormonal balance and to energize and stimulate your brain, chest, and lungs.

PRANAYAMA. During menstruation, do not practice seated pranayama or demanding or forceful breathing techniques that tighten the abdomen or challenge the nervous system. Instead practice the reclining pranayama in chapter 14 and limit it to 15 minutes.

The Days Following Menstruation

When the menstrual flow has ceased completely, introduce the inversions, that is, any of the poses described in chapter 9 that are within your practice level. Continue practicing them for three to five days following the end of menstruation. They help the organs to recover from menstruation, balance hormone levels, reestablish a balanced mental state, and prepare the body for the next cycle. Thereafter practice them at least once a week to avoid problems and to maintain health. If, during your postmenstrual phase, you participate in a regular yoga class and inversions are not included, make sure you practice them at home

The Days Leading Up to Ovulation

A woman's strength increases with rising hormone levels during the first half of the cycle. The more active poses can now be gradually introduced. I recommend that you establish a regular practice of standing poses, sitting poses, twists, backbends, and inversions. Additionally during this phase, some long, deep forward bends may provide the perfect counterbalance to rising estrogen levels.

Ovulation

At the midpoint of the cycle, a woman is at her strongest, mentally and physically. High levels of estrogen make may make tendons and ligaments more lax now, so the advanced poses are easier to perform. Be mindful to not practice with your ego. Allow common sense to guide your practice, so that you neither exploit the potential nor ignore your vulnerability.

After Ovulation

From about day nineteen or twenty, during the progesterone phase of the cycle, observe whether your energy and your ability to perform the poses changes. Some women feel progressively more sluggish as menstruation approaches. Continue with a balanced yoga practice, including standing poses, sitting poses, forward bends, inversions, back bends, and twists, throughout the remainder of the cycle, to help keep premenstrual symptoms at bay.

The Premenstrual Phase

Around the twenty-first or twenty-second day of the cycle, both progesterone and estrogen begin to decline, and the body may begin to lose elasticity. If this happens to you, take care to prepare with some warming poses prior to your back bends. The supported back bends may be good to practice now, especially if your energy is low. But don't just look at the calendar. Each woman responds in a different way to changing hormone levels. Some women become extremely flexible and supple three days before menstruation starts (hormones other than estrogen and progesterone, such as relaxin, may be at play here).

But what differentiates flexibility during the premenstrual phase from flexibility during ovulation is that there may be tendency toward inflammation. If this is the case, take special care to not overwork or tear ligaments at this time. Some women may have problems with balance. One of my students reports that in the days leading up to menstruation she has to work harder to keep Salamba Sarvangasana straight, because her hips tend to collapse to one side. For her I would recommend a supported version of the pose at this time.

Practicing the right poses at the right time is a crucial part of a woman's yoga practice. As you continue to practice yoga, you will increasingly develop awareness of your own body and its responses to the different phases of your cycle. This body awareness can give you information about when poses are good for you and when they are going against the natural flow of your energy. Listen to your own unique system, and practice using the guidelines laid out in this chapter.

Yoga as Meditation, Yoga as Prayer

The discipline of yoga promotes health and well-being, but its purpose does not end there. When a ritualized discipline, such as asana or pranayama, is part of a philosophy or religion, it has a deeper objective than strength and flexibility. It becomes a spiritual practice, which involves acknowledging, reaching out to, and aligning with forces greater than ourselves. It becomes meditation.

Yoga is meditation in action. If you organize your practice in response to all phases of your menstrual cycle, it will provide you with the power and comfort of ritual and will add stability to your life by reestablishing your link with nature's cycles. As your body takes on the forms of animals, plants, gods, and planets, yoga becomes your meditation and your prayer.

4
Starting the Journey

THE GUIDELINES in this chapter will help you prepare for a personal yoga practice. Laying claim to a place to practice is the first step. Investing in some yoga equipment is the second. (When a student tells me she doesn't want to purchase a bolster or wants to use towels instead of blankets, I know that she doesn't yet understand the importance of proper gear.)

There are many good reasons for practicing by yourself: because you like and respect yourself and because it sharpens your self-reliance. But perhaps the most important reason for practicing at home is so you can investigate your own unique hormonal patterns and observe how they play out within yourself, physically, emotionally, and spiritually. Use your personal practice, along with this book, to explore the poses and sequences that are the most relevant to your individual needs, and that help you maintain health, harmony, and balance in your life.

Before You Begin: Commonsense Advice

MEDICAL MATTERS. Sometimes menstrual and menopausal symptoms are signals of serious illness. The female reproductive system is complex and comes under all sorts of stress. This can make the uterus and accompanying parts of the body vulnerable to disease. It is imperative that you consult your medical doctor if you suffer from excessive pain, prolonged or extreme amounts of bleeding, midcycle bleeding, or bleeding with intercourse. It is also important to have regular checkups. Don't use this book or yoga alone to heal difficult conditions without getting a proper diagnosis and working along with your medical doctor's recommendations.

MOBILITY, PAIN, AND DISCOMFORT. The guidelines in this book provide clear instructions on how to practice yoga, including how not to overstretch. I show you how to differentiate between the pain that is a warning signal of an inflamed joint or an overextended muscle and the discomfort that indicates tightness that needs to be worked through. I also explain how to approach challenging poses, including cautions for each one. If you have any questions about the appropriateness of the poses or my instructions, take this book to your medical doctor for advice on how to proceed.

TEACHERS AND CLASSES. This book offers detailed instruction on using yoga to promote healthy menstrual cycles and regulate disturbances. I also recommend that you seek out a competent teacher; even one class a week will have a profound effect. If you have relatively trouble-free

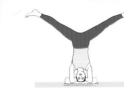

periods and are in good health, then maintain your well-being by finding a teacher you like to work with, going to regular classes, and using this book in your home practice. If you suffer from any kind of menstrual distress, such as premenstrual syndrome, menstrual cramps, or excessive bleeding, listen to your body and respond with positive action. First, consult your medical doctor, and then find an experienced teacher to work with in conjunction with this book.

Preparing for Practice

CREATING A SPACE. The first step in establishing a practice is to find a space where you can retreat and practice yoga. I live in a small apartment in New York, so I have become expert at utilizing every inch of space while respecting the needs of the people with whom I share it. With some creativity, you can make a practice space for yourself.

Of course, it's wonderful if you have a room that you can set aside for yoga. But if this is not possible, you can make do with an uncluttered area that includes a wall. The space does not have to be large, but it should be well ventilated and clean. A wooden floor is best, because wood is hard and solid and slightly porous, so it will hold your yoga mat firmly. If you must work on a carpeted floor, be sure to practice on a nonslip mat.

Most important, when you enter into your yoga space, leave behind the day's preoccupations and worries, and if possible make sure that you are not disturbed. Turn off the ringer on your telephone; remove your wristwatch; let others know that this is your practice time.

REGULAR PRACTICE. You are more likely to practice regularly if you make a schedule and maintain it. If possible, practice at the same time every day,

even if you have to cut the session a little short. That way your body and mind will establish a strong habit, and you will develop confidence by doing what you committed to do.

In Iyengar Yoga, it is customary to practice yoga for six days and to rest on the seventh, but do what works best for you. Many women work long hours outside the home, and Sundays may be the optimum time to do an extra long yoga practice. Or Sundays may be the best time to take a break from everything, including yoga. It is most important to set a realistic and sustainable goal, commit to it, and practice without disturbance.

HOW LONG? One of the main pitfalls in developing a home practice is thinking that you don't have enough time. Know this: it is always better to do something rather than nothing. If you don't have one or two hours a day for yoga, don't despair. A 10- or 15-minute practice is still a practice. Making time for yoga is part of the process of developing self-discipline. In fact, the words *practice* and *discipline* mean the same thing in this context. Regardless of how long you practice, do not rush through it. Slow down: give yourself time to explore the poses. Enjoy yourself!

TIME OF DAY. Your ability to perform the poses and the effect they have on you depends on the time of day that you practice. For example, the stimulating poses, such as unsupported back bends, may prevent you from sleeping if you practice them late in the evening, so save them for earlier in the day; mornings are most appropriate for their invigorating effect. In fact, you will sleep more soundly when you practice back bends in the morning. The seated forward bends may be easier later in the day, when your body is more flexible. Inverted poses, such as Salamba Sirsasana and Salamba Sarvangasana I and II, are best practiced later in the day, to avoid injury. If you must practice them in the morning, be sure to warm up thoroughly first.

SEQUENCING THE POSES. In addition to practicing the sequences suggested in this book, you can also make up your own. Each practice session should have a beginning, middle, and end. As a general rule, begin by waking up the body–mind with a pose like Tadasana Urdhva Hastasana. Proceed with the pose or poses that constitute the main focus of your practice that day. Complete your sequence with a resting pose.

If you are new to yoga and even if, like most women, you are flexible, do not try to master forward bends immediately. Instead, practice standing poses and relaxation poses. The standing poses will help you develop strength, stability, and hamstring elasticity. The relaxation poses will teach you how to draw quietly into yourself and will reduce fatigue.

EATING. It is a good idea to refrain from eating two hours before practicing yoga; the emptier your stomach the better. It is good to practice first thing in the morning before breakfast, and in the early evening before dinner. Allow four hours between eating a heavy meal and practicing. If you are hypoglycemic or on medication and need to eat every hour, you can practice the shorter sequences, particularly those that contain mostly restorative poses. That way, you won't have to go for hours without food. But avoid doing inversions, because in these poses even the smallest amount of food on board can cause a digestive upset. And be aware that ultimately a regular yoga practice that includes Salamba Sirsasana, Salamba Sarvanagasana I and II, and Janu Sirsasana is an excellent way of stabilizing blood sugar levels and maintaining health.

WHAT TO WEAR. Comfortable clothing that allows you to move freely, such as loose shorts and a T-shirt, is best. For a class, wear shorts with a snug band at the thigh, which are designed for optimal comfort and modesty. If you prefer something longer, tights work well, especially in classes where Iyengar Yoga teachers like to be able to see the contours of your legs. Practice with bare feet so you can spread your toes and feel your feet in contact with the floor.

The Yoga of Good Nutrition

Many students find that when they start to practice yoga they become more aware and more respectful of the body. Part of taking care of ourselves includes being sensitive to the effects of food. In terms of yoga practice, be aware of when you eat and what food you eat.

As for what you eat, here are some recommendations based on ayurvedic medicine, the ancient Indian system of preventing and healing disease. Many Western physicians are now moving closer to the ayurvedic nutritional approach, which considers that an unhealthy diet may contribute to many gynecological problems, such as fibroids, cysts, and endometriosis. The habitual consumption of coffee, diet sodas, french fries, sugar, pizzas, and fatty processed meats may cause inflammation and stagnation in the digestive system and contribute to disease, including those that affect the reproductive system. It is best to avoid heavily processed or junk foods, because they contain harmful fats and additives and few nutrients. Pesticides and chemicals used in modern farming techniques may disturb hormone balance.

If you have menstrual problems, look for any connection with the foods you eat. Keep a journal of foods consumed and note your emotions and feelings. Stress and the fast pace of life tend to

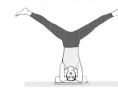

rob nutrients from the body. Your state of mind when eating is also important. Sit down quietly to eat and rest afterward, especially if you have menstrual disorders. Being overweight may contribute to hormonal imbalance and menstrual problems.

According to ayurveda, cold drinks often affect the lungs adversely and bring on coughs, congestion, and irritation, particularly around the time of menstruation, when hormone levels are low. Traditional Chinese medicine also advises against too much cold food, because it hinders movement and may cause stagnation in the body. In the same way that swimming in cold water temporarily halts the menstrual flow, cold food may restrict the movement of menstrual blood. An acupuncturist would equate dark or blackish menstrual blood or clotting with coldness in the uterus. Cramps that are relieved by a heating pad are also an indication of cold causing stagnation of the blood flow. If you suffer from such a condition, it is best to avoid cold food, such as iced drinks or ice cream, throughout the month. Just this simple dietary adjustment can make a huge difference to your menstrual symptoms.

In the five days or so leading up to your period, avoid foods high in sodium, such as processed and pickled foods, bacon, and soy sauce, especially if you are prone to premenstrual bloating. These foods may contribute to the buildup of fluid in the tissues. And you don't have to be bloated to be retaining fluid. Nausea, dizziness, feeling faint, and even problems with speech may also be symptomatic of fluid retention.

Due to the hormonal changes around the time of menstruation, blood sugar levels may become unstable, making you feel jittery and tense. Many women crave sweets at this time. Refined sugar, which can cause immune system imbalances and fatigue and may increase the symptoms of pre-

menstrual syndrome, has no nutritional value. Most nutritionists now recommend that you at least reduce the intake of refined sugar, even if you don't eliminate it completely. Alcohol also has an adverse effect on blood sugar, and it overloads the liver. A well-functioning liver is crucial for metabolizing hormones in the body. Avoid refined carbohydrates, such as white bread, white pasta, and pastries. These are converted to sugar soon after they enter your system and can contribute to yeast infections.

Premenstrual chocolate cravings may be the result of a reduction of magnesium, which often occurs around menstruation. Some nutritionists advise that you eat foods high in magnesium, such as nuts, whole grains, legumes, and vegetables, especially the leafy green kind, when these cravings arise. But if your spirit wants chocolate during times of hormonal flux, then a small amount may improve your mood. And a little high-grade dark chocolate is certainly better than reaching for pastries and doughnuts if you have premenstrual cravings.

There are healthy oils and harmful oils. It seems that most of us these days are deficient in omega-3 essential fatty acids. These essential fats help to control the fluid balance in the body and can also reduce the water retention that often occurs around the time of menstruation. Flaxseed oil, walnuts, and dark leafy greens are good sources of omega-3 essential fatty acids.

Avoid commercially produced, refined vegetable oils, such as regular sunflower oil, safflower oil (even cold-pressed), and corn oil, particularly if you suffer from endometriosis. These oils are overrefined and sometimes rancid. Also avoid all products containing hydrogenated or partially hydrogenated oils, such as artificially hardened margarine, which are particularly problematic for the immune system and may cause hardening of the arteries. Store-bought cookies and pastries, corn chips, and potato chips are just a few of the foods that usually contain these highly processed and harmful fats.

Eat foods that keep your body vital: organic, fresh vegetables and whole grains, which provide fiber and enhance colon health. Nutritionists now recommend five servings (one serving = 1½ cup) of fruit and vegetables a day. Women who eat vegetarian diets excrete more estrogen, probably because vegetarian diets tend to be higher in fiber. Organic vegetables and traditional soy products, such as tempeh, miso, tofu, natto, and edamame (green soy beans), contain phytoestrogens that are may protect against hormone-related cancers and may help balance the natural hormones in the body.

Drink plenty of fluids but avoid sweetened, caffeinated drinks. Tea, coffee, and alcohol make the nerves hypersensitive and overstimulate the adrenal glands, which can disturb the menstrual process. Nicotine has the same effect and can cause longer bleeding and menstrual cramping.

While opinions about food and diet run the gamut, one universal rule is to avoid overeating. Eat smaller amounts more frequently, especially around the time of menstruation. Never overload your plate (or anyone else's). And try to end a meal before you are stuffed full.

The foods that we eat become the physical, emotional, and spiritual aspects of our being. Home cooking, prepared by you or someone who loves you, is the best food of all. The most loving cook will create the most beneficial food. Food can be yoga, too.

Tampons

What do tampons have to do with yoga practice? you may well ask. Tampons may inhibit the flow of energy in your pelvis and therefore affect both your yoga practice and your overall health. According to some ayurvedic practitioners, tampons, which stop the menstrual flow from taking its usual path out of the vagina, also inhibit *apana*, the natural downward flow of vital energy that controls elimination.

Some women find that tampons exacerbate or even cause menstrual cramps, and that discomfort goes away if they switch to pads. And most worryingly, tampons are a suspected cause of some serious gynecological diseases. The use of tampons has been implicated in the development of endometriosis, fibroids, and the formation of cysts. The super-absorbent kind of tampon that contains a high percentage of rayon has been linked with the relatively rare but potentially life-threatening toxic shock syndrome. (There are also other factors that play into these conditions, such as poor nutrition and stress, both of which compromise the immune system.) Tampons often contain bleached paper that has been exposed to the carcinogenic chemical dioxin, which is released as a byproduct of the bleaching process. Tampon manufacturers are not required by law to state the ingredients in their products, so unless you choose a tampon brand that lists the ingredients, it is impossible to know exactly what you are using.

Of course tampons are convenient and give many women a sense of freedom, so it is unlikely that we will all decide to give them up. If we use common sense, we can minimize the risks of tampon use. There is no doubt that bacteria can grow on a tampon, particularly if it is left in for too long. One of my yoga student reports that she develops a painful rash in and around the vagina if she uses tampons at night, when it is worn for eight hours or longer.

If you choose to wear tampons, wear the very best you can. Minimize the adverse effects by

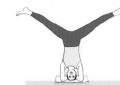

using those that are unbleached, chemical-free, 100 percent cotton. Change your tampon at least every four to six hours, and consider converting to menstrual pads at night and on light days.

Supporting Your Practice: Using Props

A fascinating and important aspect of B. K. S. Iyengar's pioneering work is yoga therapy, which includes the innovative use of props. Unlike the gleaming space-age machinery of elaborately equipped sports clubs, yoga props may seem rather low-tech. But the ideas and concepts behind their use are sophisticated and profoundly effective. Used sensitively and intelligently, props can enhance yoga practice. Equipment as simple as a wooden block, a bolster, or a chair can be used to stretch, suspend, fold, or twist the body into a healing response.

For yoga to be effective, it is important to stay in the poses for a while. However, there are times, such as during menstruation, when energy may be low and when the sheer effort of holding a posture can negate its benefits. With the help of props, you can stay in a pose longer, find your alignment, and really listen to what your body is telling you. By working with the support of something as simple as a chair or a wall, you can overcome weakness and conserve energy. When there is stiffness or tightness in the joints or spine, prop support allows you to work through and release rigidity without fear of injury. A pose can also be more challenging and more deeply understood through the use of props. For example, practicing Viparita Dandasana II with Arms Through Chair will leave you free to concentrate on the coiling action of your upper back.

The Woman's Yoga Book PROP KIT. Here are the props that you will need to practice with this book. You can get them from the suppliers listed in resources.

4.1

1 NONSLIP MAT

Dimensions: 68" x 24"

Alternative: wood or linoleum floor

There are many nonslip mats on the market; choose whichever you prefer. More experienced students can sometimes work without a mat because they can "hold" the floor with their feet in standing poses.

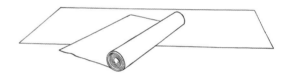

4.2

5 OR 6 BLANKETS

Dimensions (unfolded): 55" x 85"

Alternative: twin size blankets

Blankets used for yoga should provide a firm support and should be identical. They should be of good quality and not be too spongy, slippery, bulky, or thin. Blankets made of mixed cotton and acrylic work well because of their compact weave and their thickness. Alternatively you can use 100 percent wool or cotton.

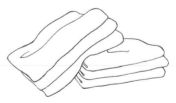

第6贴　反面 凯源–4色–WomandYoga–内页拼版．job

4·3
1 OR 2 ROUND BOLSTERS

Dimensions: 26" long x 32" circumference
Alternative: Roll three blankets into a cylindrical shape and secure with one or two yoga straps.

Bolsters are an important investment for yoga because they provide firm support for the poses that are so important to practice during menstruation. When reclining over a bolster, the body molds itself to the cylindrical shape, effecting a horizontal and vertical stretch. This "opens" the chest or pelvis as it conserves energy.

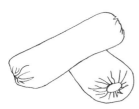

4·4
2 FOLDING CHAIRS

Dimensions: Chair seat approximately 16" x 16"
Alternative: sturdy chairs without casters

Use a regular wooden (or metal) folding chair with enough space between the seat and the backrest (at least 11") so you can climb through it. Make sure the chair is heavy enough to not tip over when you climb through or over it.

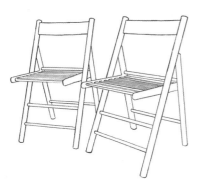

4·5
2 BLOCKS

Dimensions: 9" x 5" x 3½"
Alternative: books tied or taped together

It is important to have two identical blocks. They can be made of foam or wood. Telephone books are also useful; stabilize them with two pieces of cardboard, cut to the dimensions of the book, placed over the front and back covers. Bind the whole package with heavy tape.

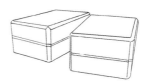

4·6
2 STRAPS

Dimensions: 1" x 75"
Alternative: bathrobe tie

Of all the straps now on the market, the best one is the Pune Belt, which was designed by B. K. S. Iyengar. It is cotton, with a sliding bar. It is the most efficient and trouble-free method of securing your poses. Alternatively you can use any belt offered by yoga suppliers.

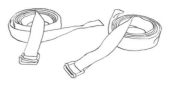

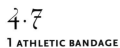

4.7

¶ ATHLETIC BANDAGE

Dimensions: 4½" x 100"

Alternative: Small folded towel or washcloth

The bandage is used to cover the eyes or to wrap around the head. It helps you to be less distracted and to focus inward and relax more deeply during a restorative or pranayama practice. It is particularly helpful if you have a migraine headache or insomnia.

4.8

¶ SANDBAG

Dimensions: Approximately 19" x 9"; 10–15 pounds

Alternative: a 10-pound bag of rice or kitty litter

In this book, a sandbag is placed across the thighs in Savasana to relieve the lower back. Alternatively you can place a bolster and some folded blankets across your thighs for a similar effect.

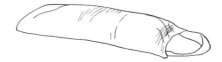

4.9

TELEPHONE BOOKS

This prop is useful for when you need to add height, such as in Kapotasana (see 10.5d), or in instead of blocks (see description for block alternative in this chapter).

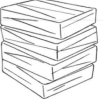

4.10

¶ TIMER, WATCH, OR CLOCK

This aid is good for the times when you need to watch the clock and you don't want to have to! When practicing Salamba Sirasaana turn your wristwatch on its side and place it in front of you where you can see it. You can set your timer or watch to beep at the end of Savasana.

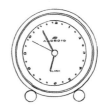

To best prepare for yoga practice, honor your body and your soul by listening to them. Make a pleasant, private, peaceful space in which to practice. Buy good-quality props and assemble what you need for the day's practice. Eat healthily, keep regular hours, and follow those pursuits that make you happy. In this way you will successfully integrate yoga into your life.

Onward to the asana and pranayama practices. Chapters 5 through 11 take you through all the major categories of yoga poses, from standing poses to pranayama. The value of yoga depends on the level of awareness and precision that you bring to it. Following the guidelines given in these chapters will enable you to find the basic structure of the pose and then to refine your actions within the pose.

Make sure you read all the way through the instructions for each pose before practicing the sequences. And feel free to refer back to them any time you need refresh your memory. Pay particular attention to the cautions given at the end of each description of the main pose, in case you should be practicing it for medical reasons. The cautions will also tell you if this is a pose you should not do while menstruating.

About language: Each school of yoga has developed its own vocabulary, and yoga in the style of B. K. S. Iyengar is no different. Some of the phrases that I use to describe how to work in the poses or various areas of the body may sound unusual. But as you practice and make the poses your own, directions such as "lift the thigh muscles" and "firm your kneecaps" will begin to make perfect sense.

第7贴　正面 凯源-4色-WomandYoga-内页拼版.job

5

Standing Poses and a Flowing Sequence: Building a Support System

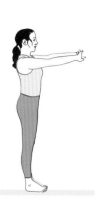

S TANDING POSES are the basis of Iyengar Yoga. Their practice should be firmly established before exploring the more advanced poses, and thereafter they should be maintained as part of your regular practice. Standing poses build strong healthy bones, remove stiffness in the joints and spine, and improve muscle tone. They improve circulation, help to maintain a healthy digestive function, strengthen the nervous system, and help develop stamina. They also teach us alignment.

Bad posture is brought about by physical weakness and mental tiredness. When the upper back becomes stooped and rounded, the chest compresses, and the heart and lungs don't function as well as they could. Bad posture can also adversely affect the function of the abdominal organs; for example, wearing high-heeled shoes shifts weight to the toes and throws the body weight forward onto the abdomen. This eventually causes the lower back and pelvic floor to weaken and strains the internal organs. Practiced correctly, the standing poses contribute to a healthy posture, whether standing, sitting, or walking, and enhance well-being. The spine is stabilized and, without sucking in or tensing the stomach, the organs are held in proper alignment. This helps guard against pelvic inflammations,

disorders of the reproductive organs, and menstrual problems.

General Cautions for Practicing the Standing Poses and Vinyasa

When practicing the standing poses and flowing sequence presented in this chapter, remember to follow these guidelines. Cautions are also included with each pose.

- The breath is an integral part of all asana practice. It should flow easily and effortlessly throughout the duration of your practice of the standing poses. If your breath becomes labored, come out of the pose and rest in Uttanasana or one of its modifications. In general, move into a pose, or make your adjustments within a pose, on an exhalation. Do not hold your breath.

- If you have high blood pressure, glaucoma, a heart condition, a headache, or an overactive thyroid, practice only the supported standing poses.

- All unsupported standing poses and most of supported poses are contraindicated during menstruation because they disturb the *apana vayu*, which is the energy in the pelvis that governs downward movement.

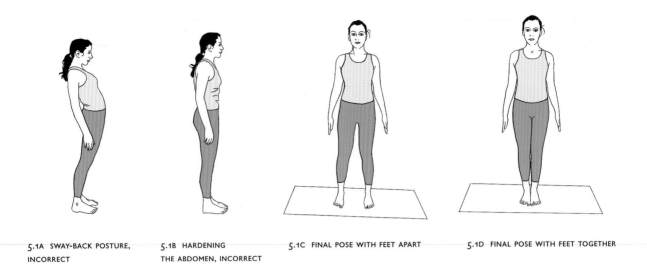

■ If you are including the two supported standing poses that can be practiced during menstruation, do not jump into them. Step your feet apart instead.

5.1

Tadasana
Mountain Pose

BENEFITS. Tadasana teaches the art of standing and taking your place in the world. Having your feet planted firmly on the ground creates emotional and physical stability and brings tremendous peace of mind. Tadasana also helps alleviate disorders caused by faulty posture. Standing with the feet splayed out, for example, creates abdominal distortion and stresses the spine. A swayback (what I call a permanent little-girl posture) weakens the spine and pushes the stomach forward, placing pressure on the uterus, ovaries, and pelvic floor (5.1a). Sucking the stomach in and compressing the pelvic muscles is equally hard on the female organs; a hard, flat stomach is just as unhealthy for women as a stomach that is weak or protruding (5.1b).

When a woman holds herself erect and without strain, she is rewarded not only with the outward signs of grace and beauty but with healthy organs, a smoothly running nervous system, hormonal equilibrium, and vitality.

PRACTICE. Stand on your mat, with your feet hip-width apart and the outer edges of your feet parallel (5.1c). Feel the soles of your feet in complete contact with the floor. Balance your body weight evenly between both feet. Lift and spread your toes and lengthen them from the base to the tips, and then allow them to rest lightly on the floor. Draw the arches of your feet and your inner ankle bones up.

Bring your legs to life by pulling your kneecaps back into the knee joints and lifting the thigh muscles. Shift your weight back a little by rolling onto your heels. This creates an important foundation from which to align your pelvis.

In Tadasana, it is important to keep your abdomen soft and the organs aligned within the pelvis. Move your tailbone into the pelvis, bring the top of your pubic bone in and up, and lift your chest, without throwing your thighs or pelvis forward.

Opening the chest helps to free the emotional center that lies just behind the breastbone. Release your shoulder blades down and away from your neck, and press them forward and onto your back ribs. Lengthen through the crown of

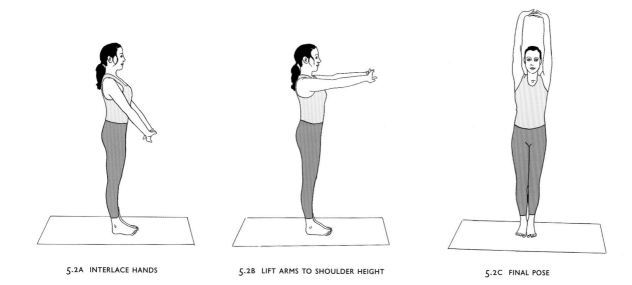

5.2A INTERLACE HANDS   5.2B LIFT ARMS TO SHOULDER HEIGHT   5.2C FINAL POSE

your head. Raise your chest and lift your breast-bone. Extend your arms down by your sides, lining up your middle fingers with the center of your outer thighs. Relax your throat, eyes, and tongue.

Repeat Tadasana, this time with your feet together (5.1d). If you are practicing with your feet apart, step them together to come out of the pose.

CAUTIONS. Do not practice Tadasana longer than 30 seconds if you have low blood pressure. Do not practice with your feet together during menstruation.

5.2
Tadasana Urdhva Baddhangullyasana
Mountain Pose with Upward-Facing Interlocked Hands

BENEFITS. Although relatively simple in appearance, Tadasana Urdhva Baddhangullyasana has dramatic effects. It improves posture, exercises the hands and knuckles, improves mobility in the shoulder joints, and boosts the circulation around the breasts.

PRACTICE. Stand on your mat in Tadasana, feet together (5.1d). Interlace your hands, and turn your palms down and away from you, so you are looking at the backs of your hands (5.2a). Exhale and lift your arms until they are at shoulder height (5.2b). Roll your shoulders back and press your hands away from you. Inhale and, maintaining the steadiness of your legs, lift your arms up and over your head (5.2c).

Straighten your arms by pulling your elbows in and toward each other. Press the knuckles of your index fingers toward the ceiling. Do not allow your thighs or lower ribs to project forward.

To change sides, bring your hands down until they are level with your shoulders. Turn your palms toward you. Change the interlock of your fingers, so the opposite thumb is on top. Turn the palms away from you, and swing your arms overhead.

To come out, lower your interlocked hands to shoulder height. Roll your shoulders back and press your hands away from you. Turn your palms toward you and release the interlock. Lower your arms to your sides.

CAUTIONS. If you suffer from hypertension, do not lift your arms overhead in this or any other pose. Do not practice this pose if you have a migraine or are suffering from insomnia.

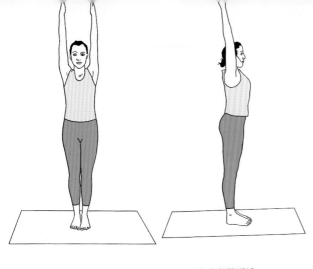

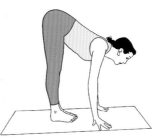

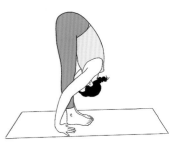

5.3A FINAL POSE

5.4A ARMS OVERHEAD,
PALMS FORWARD

5.4B RAISE HEAD, LOOK UP

5.4C FINAL POSE

5·3
Tadasana Urdhva Hastasana
Mountain Pose with Arms Overhead

BENEFITS. In addition to the benefits of Tadasana, this pose relieves stiffness in the shoulder joints, tones and stimulates the abdomen and spine, and counteracts depression.

PRACTICE. Stand in Tadasana, feet together (5.1d). With your arms facing each other and without throwing your thighs forward, inhale and swing your arms forward and up over your head (5.3a). Straighten your arms and extend through your fingers. Firm your shoulder blades into your back. The upper arms should be in line with your ears. If your hands are forward of your head, then press your shoulder blades more firmly against your rib cage and move your arms back. To come out, exhale and swing your arms forward and down.

CAUTIONS. Do not practice this pose if you are suffering from migraine headache or hypertension.

5·4
Uttanasana
Standing Forward Bend Pose

BENEFITS. Compression around the abdomen can restrict blood flow around the uterus, ovaries, and fallopian tubes. Uttanasana releases tension in the abdomen and helps to prevent the buildup of fatty deposits in the area. It also massages the internal organs, which in turn influences the ovaries and helps establish a healthy menstrual cycle. The first stage of this pose, where head and trunk are lifted, is particularly beneficial for women, because it helps to release abdominal tension and may also relieve abdominal cramps. The final pose, where the head is down, relieves backache, constipation, and stiffness in the spine, neck, and shoulders. In addition, blood flow to the breasts is stimulated. But the most immediate benefit of Uttanasana, and perhaps the one we are the most grateful for, is the softening of the facial muscles and the calming effect it has on the brain.

PRACTICE. Stand on your mat in Tadasana, feet together (5.1d). Inhale and raise your hands overhead, with your palms facing forward (5.4a). Exhale and bend forward. Place your fingertips

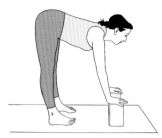

5.4D WITH BLOCKS IN FRONT OF FEET

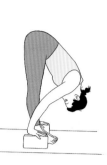

5.4E WITH BLOCKS AT SIDES OF FEET

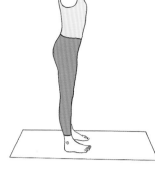

5.4F SWING FOLDED ARMS OVERHEAD

5.4G WITH ARMS FOLDED

on the floor in front of you. Raise your head and look up (5.4b).

Firm your kneecaps onto the knee joints and draw your thigh muscles up. Extend your rib cage and breastbone forward, and curve your spine in. If you are very flexible, take care not to push the lumbar spine down onto your belly. Move your shoulder blades away from your neck. Roll forward onto the front of your feet until your legs are perpendicular to the floor. Then take the head and trunk down: Without losing the extension of the abdomen, lift the sitting bones up and away from the backs of the thighs and roll them out and away from the tailbone; fold your trunk forward and down. Slide your hands back to rest at the sides of your feet (5.4c). Allow your front ribs to lengthen and your jaw and eyes to relax.

To come out, move into the concave position again: Pull your torso forward and up. Raise your head and look up. Place your hands on your hips. Inhale and stand up. Return to Tadasana.

CAUTIONS. Do not practice the final position, with the head down, if you have a herniated disk. If the pose causes dizziness, make sure you are warmed up (by practicing some standing poses), and if that does not help, then practice Uttanasana with Head Support (5.4h) or Uttanasana with Wall and Chair (5.4i) instead. Avoid it completely dur-

ing menstruation if you have low blood pressure or feel fatigued.

UTTANASANA WITH BLOCKS. If you cannot reach the floor with your hands without bending your knees or rounding your back, place your hands on blocks. Make sure you do not lean into or away from the blocks. Start with the blocks in front of your feet when stretching your spine forward (5.4d). In the head down position, slide the blocks to the sides of your feet (5.4e).

UTTANASANA WITH ARMS FOLDED. Here is another alternative if you cannot place your hands on the floor. Practice it also to rest between standing poses. Stand in Tadasana with the feet apart (5.1c). Fold your arms and hold your elbows. Inhale and swing them above your head (5.4f). Exhale and fold forward from the hips (5.4g). Allow the weight of the elbows to release your side body down. When ready change the grip of the elbows and repeat. To come out, release your elbows. Place your hands on your hips, inhale, and bring your head up first.

UTTANASANA WITH HEAD SUPPORT. Often during menstruation, it is hard to concentrate. This variation enables the brain to recover from mental fatigue, restores mental clarity, and can be held

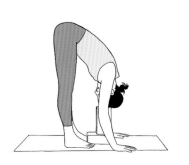

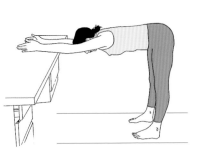

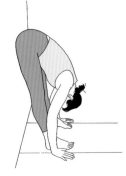

5.4H WITH HEAD SUPPORT

5.4I WITH WALL AND CHAIR

5.4J ARDHA UTTANASANA WITH ARMS ON COUNTERTOP OR CHAIR

5.4K PARSVA UTTANASANA WITH WALL, ROLL DOWN FROM WAIST

for a longer time. It reduces high blood pressure, lowers the heart rate, and has a soothing effect on the nervous system. It also relieves lower back pain.

Place one or more blocks in front of you on your mat. The height of your support depends on your body proportions and flexibility. Stand in Tadasana, facing the block or blocks, with your feet about 1 foot apart (5.1c). Place your hands on your hips, exhale, and curving your spine in and leading with your breastbone, bend forward. Place the top of your head on the block (5.4h), without compressing your neck or bending your legs. Fully stretch your legs. Relax your eyes, throat, and tongue.

UTTANASANA WITH WALL AND CHAIR. Practice this variation if tight hamstrings and stiff hips will not allow your head to reach the blocks. Stand a chair on a mat, the short end of which touches the wall. Place a folded blanket on the seat. Lean against a wall and position your feet to the edges of the mat. Bend forward and place your head on the chair seat. (If your head does not reach, place a bolster across the seat). Thread your arms through the chair, palms facing, and stretch them away from you (5.4i). Slide your sit bones farther up the wall. Keep your feet active; spread the toes. Extend out through your fingers and draw your

arm muscles back toward your shoulders. Feel the heaviness of the brain where the head touches the chair and relax your face, eyes, and tongue. Breathe easily and evenly.

ARDHA UTTANASANA WITH ARMS ON COUNTERTOP OR CHAIR. Particularly helpful when tension causes the menstrual flow to become excessive or light, or when menstruation is delayed, this modification also helps to remove premenstrual tightness in the abdomen, upper back, and shoulders. Stand on your mat in Tadasana, feet apart (5.1c). Place your hands on your hips, exhale and bend forward, keeping your legs straight. Extend your arms out in front of you, with your palms facing in, and place your outer wrists on the top of a countertop or chair back (5.4j). Straighten your elbows and extend through your fingertips. Firm your kneecaps and draw your thigh muscles up toward the pelvis. Keep the arches of the feet active. Take care not to sink into the abdomen. Maintain an even extension along the length of the spine.

PARSVA UTTANASANA WITH WALL. This pose cools the body and soothes the muscles along the sides of the lumbar spine. Always follow unsupported backbends with this pose.

Place the short end of your mat against the

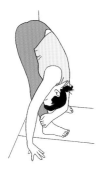

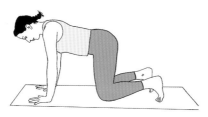

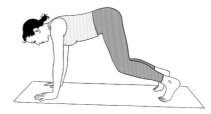

5.4L PARSVA UTTANASANA
WITH WALL, FINAL POSE

5.5A KNEEL DOWN

5.5B TURN TOES UNDER

wall. Place your buttocks against the wall and your feet a little more than hip-width apart. With your hands on your hips, exhale and slowly roll down from the waist (5.4k). Notice the width of the sacrum and the broadness of the lumbar as you bend forward and release your head and torso down. Slide your torso to the right. Hold your outer right ankle with your left hand, and place your right hand on the floor by the side of your right foot (5.4l). Descend the crown of your head toward the floor.

Return to the center and repeat the pose to the other side. To come out, inhale and slowly roll up to Tadasana, lifting your head last, and step away from the wall. Do not practice this pose if you have bulging or herniated disks or low blood pressure.

5.5
Adho Mukha Svanasana
Downward-Facing Dog Pose

BENEFITS. If you have time to practice only one pose, make it Adho Mukha Svanasana, because it combines many of the elements of the standing poses. The wrists, arms, and legs are strengthened. Flexibility is improved in the shoulders and hips. This pose also provides traction for the spine, rests the heart, and restores energy. It increases the circulation around the breasts and abdomen and helps keep constipation at bay. It also helps to correct a displaced uterus. Practice Adho Mukha Svanasana regularly between your periods to prevent menstrual headaches and to help the glands function properly when menstruation comes around.

PRACTICE. Kneel on your mat, with your hands on the floor, slightly forward of your shoulders, and your knees directly under your hips (5.5a). Spread your palms. Turn your toes under and raise your knees off the floor (5.5b). Exhale and swing back onto the balls of your feet (5.5c).

Secure the base of the pose. Press your index finger knuckles down and extend through your

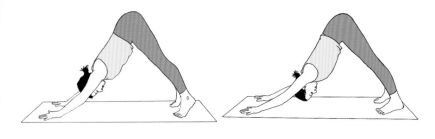

5.5C SWING ONTO BALLS OF FEET   5.5D FINAL POSE

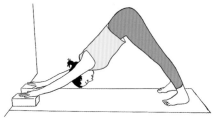

5.5E WITH BLOCKS AGAINST WALL

fingers. Broaden across the balls of your feet and extend your toes forward. Press your thighs and shinbones back. Lift your kneecaps and sitting bones, and descend your heels toward the floor (5.5d).

Keeping your elbows stable, fully extend your arms away from your hands. Pull your deltoids into your shoulder blades, and draw your shoulder blades away from your neck. Maintain an even extension along the left and right sides of your torso and armpits.

With continued practice, your hamstrings will lengthen and your spine will release, and Adho Mukha Svanasana can be done without the belly getting sucked toward the lower back.

To come out, lower your knees to the floor and sit in Virasana (6.8c). Alternatively, step forward into Uttanasana (5.4c), that is, bring your feet in between your hands, and rest for a few breaths. When you are ready, place your hands on your hips, inhale, and come to Tadasana, feet together.

CAUTIONS. Do not practice Adho Mukha Svanasana or its modifications if you have a headache or diarrhea. Consult an experienced yoga teacher and your health care practitioner if you have wrist problems or carpal tunnel syndrome.

ADHO MUKHA SVANASANA WITH BLOCKS OR CHAIR AGAINST WALL. If your shoulders are stiff, prop your hands on blocks (5.5e) or on a chair seat (5.5f) to facilitate an easier stretch through the shoulders. What you need depends on your flexibility.

ADHO MUKHA SVANASANA WITH HEAD SUPPORT. This modification is safe for those with high blood pressure. However, be sensitive to how you feel. Do not practice it if you experience ringing in your ears, dizziness, or pounding or pressure in your head.

If you are very flexible, this pose will help avoid overarching the lumbar spine and pushing down onto the abdomen, a movement that is particularly stressful to the uterus and weakening for the low back. It also helps relieve the heaviness and fatigue of bloating in the thighs and pelvis during the premenstrual phase, and it quiets the brain. You can hold the pose longer when the head is supported.

Place your mat with the short end touching the wall. Place two blocks, shoulder-width apart, with the short ends against the wall. Position one or more blocks about 21 inches from the wall for your head. The prop height that you need depends on your flexibility.

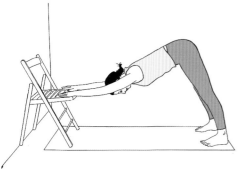

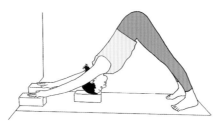

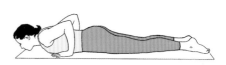

5.5F WITH CHAIR AGAINST WALL   5.5G WITH HEAD SUPPORT   5.6A DRAW ELBOWS TOWARD SIDE RIBS

Kneel down, facing the wall. Place your hands on the blocks, the heel of the hand braced against the front edge. Raise your knees and stretch your legs back. Fully stretch your arms, then exhale and, without shortening the neck or bending the elbows or legs, place your head on the block (5.5g). Come down and adjust the prop height if necessary.

Move the inner edges of the shoulder blades into your back and away from your neck. Draw your outer hipbones back so your torso and armpits lengthen.

Come down and rest for a few breaths in Adho Mukha Virasana (6.9c) before standing up. Return to Tadasana, feet together.

5.6

Urdhva Mukha Svanasana
Upward-Facing Dog Pose

BENEFITS. Urdhva Mukha Svanasana strengthens the upper body, creates mobility in the spine, and stimulates the thyroid gland.

PRACTICE. Lie face down on your mat, with your feet hip-width apart and your toes facing straight back. Place your hands on the floor on either side of your rib cage, with your fingers pointing forward. Draw your elbows in toward your side ribs (5.6a).

With an inhalation, raise your head and chest and, straightening your arms, lift the pelvis and thighs off the floor (5.6b). Draw your kneecaps firmly into the knee joints. Swing your upper torso through your arms, and allow the weight of the body to be evenly distributed between the palms of the hands and the tops of the feet (5.6c).

Press your hands down and release your shoulders away from your ears. Move your upper arms back and turn them out. Press your inner elbows forward. Lengthen your spine from the front of

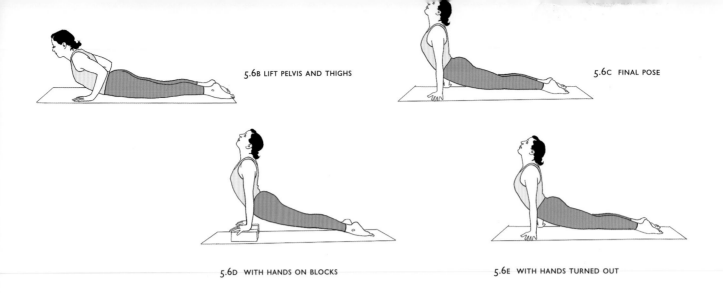

5.6B LIFT PELVIS AND THIGHS

5.6C FINAL POSE

5.6D WITH HANDS ON BLOCKS

5.6E WITH HANDS TURNED OUT

your tailbone, and lift the sides of your chest. Firm your buttock muscles and tuck your tailbone in. Raise your inner thighs away from the floor.

To avoid straining the abdominal area, arch your spine evenly along its length. Coil your shoulder blades onto your back ribs. Lift and broaden your chest even more, and spread your collarbones. Curve your upper torso up and back until your breastbone faces the ceiling. Don't compress your neck. Release your shoulders away from the neck, move your head back, and look up.

With an exhalation, lower your torso to the floor. Release your arms to the sides. Turn onto your right side. Press your left hand into the floor and push up to sitting, bringing the head up last.

CAUTION. Do not practice this pose or the modifications during menstruation.

URDHVA MUKHA SVANASANA WITH HANDS ON BLOCKS. If your arms are weak and you cannot lift your thighs off the floor, place your hands on blocks (5.6d).

URDHVA MUKHA SVANASANA WITH HANDS TURNED OUT. If your wrists, elbows, or shoulders are weak, practice with the hands turned out (5.6e).

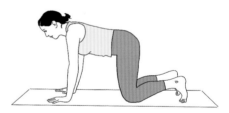

5.7A METHOD 1: BEGIN ON ALL FOURS

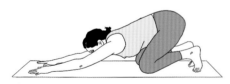

5.7B METHOD 1: HIPS ON HEELS

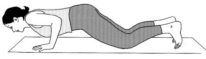

5.7C METHOD 1: LOWER TORSO

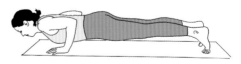

5.7D FINAL POSE

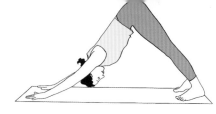

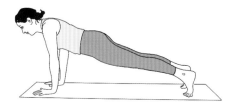

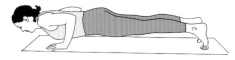

5·7

Chaturanga Dandasana
Plank Pose

BENEFITS. Most of the women who come to my beginners' class find Chaturanga Dandasana almost impossible at the outset. But after a few months of concerted effort, their upper bodies become robust and strong. Even those who lift weights at the gym find that this pose is by far the most effective method of strengthening the arms and shoulders. Chaturanga Dandasana tones and strengthens the upper body and develops abdominal strength. Additionally, it helps prepare for Salamba Sirsasana (9.2d), Salamba Sarvangasana I (9.3f), and backbends.

PRACTICE. Here are two methods of coming into the pose. Begin by working with whichever method gets you into the pose with the most ease.

METHOD 1: This method may be easier for women. Kneel down with your hips directly over your knees and your hands a little forward of your shoulders (5.7a). Tuck your toes under. Spread your fingers and press the knuckles of your index fingers down. Drop your hips back onto your heels (5.7b). Roll your shoulders back, and firm your shoulder blades into your back ribs. Keeping your head and shoulders close to the floor, exhale and propel your torso forward and down to about 5 inches from the floor (5.7c). Inhale, raise your knees off the floor, and straighten your legs. Look ahead (5.7d).

METHOD 2: Begin in Adho Mukha Svanasana (5.7e). Keeping your arms straight, exhale and swing your torso forward, bringing your shoulders directly above your wrists (5.7f). Exhale again, bend your elbows back, and lower yourself to within 5 inches of the floor. Fully straighten your legs. Look ahead (5.7g).

Drop your pelvis until it is level with your shoulders. The underside of the body should align evenly above the floor. Extend your heels back, so your feet are vertical. Stretch and open the back of your knees, and draw your kneecaps up into the knee joint. Raise your inner thighs toward the ceiling. Holding your legs and heels firm, move your rib cage and collarbones forward toward your head and roll your shoulders back. Keep your upper arms connected into your upper back; that is, move your shoulder blades away from your neck. Breathe evenly.

Exhale and release down to the floor. Bring your arms to your sides. Roll onto your side and

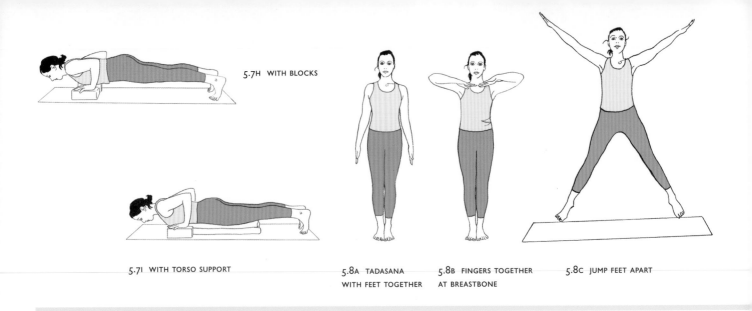

5.7H WITH BLOCKS

5.7I WITH TORSO SUPPORT

5.8A TADASANA
WITH FEET TOGETHER

5.8B FINGERS TOGETHER
AT BREASTBONE

5.8C JUMP FEET APART

rest for a few breaths. Push up from your hands to come up to sitting.

CAUTIONS. This pose is strenuous and should not be practiced during menstruation or if you have had recent abdominal surgery. Avoid it altogether if you have fibroid tumors, endometriosis, ovarian cysts, or if you suffer from an excessively heavy menstrual flow.

CHATURANGA DANDASANA WITH BLOCKS. If you experience difficulty lifting yourself off the floor, support your hands on blocks (5.7h).

CHATURANGA DANDASANA WITH TORSO SUPPORT. If you need more support, prop your torso on one or more folded blankets (5.7i). Practice with props until you have gained the strength to do the pose unsupported.

5.8
Jumping from Tadasana to Utthita Hasta Padasana
Jumping the Legs Apart

BENEFITS. Jumping is the quickest and most efficient way of landing with equal weight on both

feet. It also energizes and stimulates the cardio-vascular system.

PRACTICE. Stand on your mat in Tadasana, feet together (5.8a). Bend your elbows and bring your fingertips together at the breastbone (5.8b). Inhale deeply, sweep your arms out to the sides, and at the same time jump your feet so they land 4 feet apart. Keep your arms at shoulder height and your palms turned down. As you jump, open and lift your ribs (5.8c). Maintain this lift as you land in Utthita Hasta Padasana (5.8d). Look to see that the outer edges of your feet are parallel. If necessary, reposition them. Jump your feet back to Tadasana.

CAUTIONS. Do not jump into poses if you have a herniated disk, sciatica, knee or ankle problems, or are menstruating.

5.9
Utthita Trikonasana
Extended Triangle Pose

BENEFITS. Utthita Trikonasana strengthens the legs and arms, mobilizes the spine and neck, and increases the circulation to the hip and shoulder

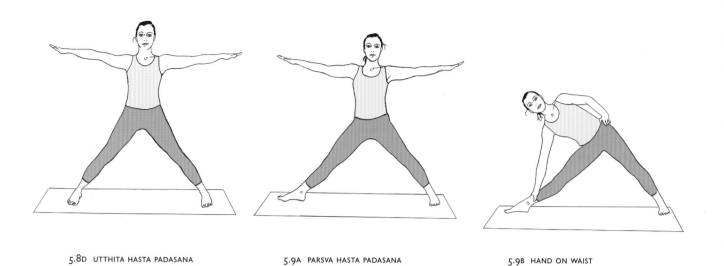

5.8D UTTHITA HASTA PADASANA   5.9A PARSVA HASTA PADASANA   5.9B HAND ON WAIST

joints. For some, it can also relieve backache and menstrual cramps. In addition this pose tones the internal organs, improves digestion and elimination, and reduces menstrual disorders.

PRACTICE. Stand on the mat in Tadasana, feet together (5.8a). With an exhalation, jump (or step) your feet 4 feet apart into Utthita Hasta Padasana (5.8d). Extend out through your fingertips and straighten your elbows. Draw your shoulder blades down and lift your chest up. Straighten your legs by drawing your knees and thighs up.

Turn your right leg and foot out 90 degrees. Come into Parsva Hasta Padasana by pivoting on your left heel and turning your left foot in (5.9a). Align your right heel with the arch of your left foot. Spread your toes and hold the floor well with the soles of your feet. As you turn your feet to the right, turn your pelvis to the left, away from your right leg, so your navel faces straight ahead and is aligned with your breastbone.

With an exhalation, extend your torso to the right and drop your right hand onto your right shinbone. Place your left hand on your waist. Turn your chest toward the ceiling and look straight ahead (5.9b).

Press down through the inner edge of the right foot. Simultaneously, turn the right thigh out and pull the right kneecap up. Lengthen down through the core of your left leg, and press your outer left heel down. Move your pelvis forward to align it directly above the invisible line that runs between your feet. Move your upper torso back to align it directly above your pelvis and feet.

Lengthen through your spine by drawing your tailbone toward your left heel and extending the right side of your torso away from your right hip. If you feel that your spine is not fully extended, come up and move your back foot away from the forward foot, and come down again.

Roll your left shoulder back. Draw the muscles of your upper back into your back ribs, and sink your right shoulder blade into your body. Raise your left arm. Open the right side of your chest toward the ceiling. Straighten your right arm and turn your right inner elbow out. Look up and gaze at your left thumbnail with quiet eyes (5.9c). Relax your throat. Breathe!

Provided that you are not menstruating, you can keep your arms lifted as you change sides. This is hard work but it helps to build upper body strength and develop stamina. Press down into your back foot and inhale as you come up. Turn your feet to the front, then to the other side, and repeat the pose. When you have done the pose to both sides, turn your feet to the front and step or jump your feet back to Tadasana.

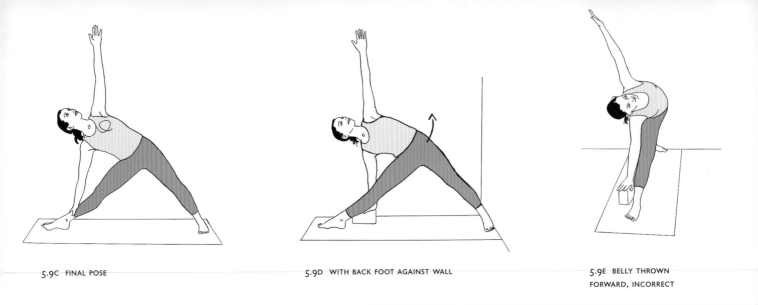

5.9C FINAL POSE   5.9D WITH BACK FOOT AGAINST WALL   5.9E BELLY THROWN FORWARD, INCORRECT

CAUTIONS. Do not practice this pose unsupported during menstruation. Wait for three days following menstruation to resume practice of this pose.

UTTHITA TRIKONASANA WITH BACK FOOT AGAINST WALL.

This modification benefits women, because bracing the back leg against the wall provides a secure framework from which to align and adjust the pelvis.

To practice, place the short side of your mat against the wall and your block at the opposite end of the mat to support your right hand. Stand on the mat with your left shoulder toward the wall. Place your left hand on the wall, at shoulder height, and position your outer left foot against the wall. Step your right foot out approximately 4 feet. Raise your right arm to shoulder height, palm down. Turn your right foot out, keeping the heel of the right foot in line with the arch of the left. Exhale and extend your torso to the right and place your right hand on the block (5.9d).

Focus on supporting the abdominal organs. Align your pelvis over the midline that runs between your feet. Coil your right buttock firmly onto your right buttock bone. Press the soles of your feet into the floor and, keeping your legs straight, turn your pelvis, waist, and chest to the left.

If you allow your lower spine to sag and throw the belly forward (5.9e, incorrect), or conversely if you harden the belly against your lower back or push the pelvis back (5.9f, incorrect), the resulting abdominal tension may irritate your uterus. Use your tailbone to help you gently guide the top of your pubic bone into the pelvis and up. Open your left hipbone away from your right hip joint. Move the top of your left thigh back to line up with the midline (5.9g, correct). Notice the feeling of support that comes to the belly. Fully open the chest.

UTTHITA TRIKONASANA WITH WALL AND BLOCK.

Practicing with your back against the wall enables you to align the pelvis and shoulders over the feet more easily. Also the wall support helps you focus on other aspects of the pose, such as opening the chest and lengthening the lumbar spine to relieve abdominal or lower back pain. Working this way is helpful for those with high blood pressure and is safe to practice during menstruation, because the support takes some of the effort out of the pose.

Place the long side of your mat against the wall. Stand with your back to the wall. Come into the pose, with your right hand supported on a block. Do not let the lumbar spine fall away from the

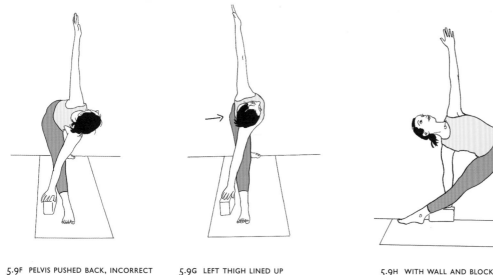

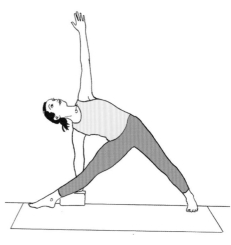

5.9F PELVIS PUSHED BACK, INCORRECT

5.9G LEFT THIGH LINED UP WITH MIDLINE, CORRECT

5.9H WITH WALL AND BLOCK

wall, because doing so places strain on the internal organs. Roll your left hip and shoulder back to the wall. Straighten your legs and arms (5.9h).

If you have an overactive thyroid, you can practice this modification, but look down toward the floor or straight ahead to avoid overexerting or overstimulating the gland.

UTTITHA TRIKONASANA FACING WALL. If you have soreness or bloating in the abdomen, practice facing the wall. This pose helps reduce irritations and inflammations of the pelvic organs and benefits those with fibroids, ovarian cysts, or scar tissue, because you can more easily draw the pelvic organs back to their proper place, and healing takes place when the body is aligned correctly.

Place the long side of your mat against the wall. Stand facing the wall, with your legs 4 feet apart and turned to the right. Come into Utthita Trikonasana, with your right hand supported on a block that has been placed beside your outer right ankle. Place your left hand on the wall (5.9i). Lengthen your tailbone away from your head, and coil your right buttock onto your right buttock bone and toward the wall. Roll your left hipbone to the left, away from the wall. Draw your frontal hipbones up, toward your chest. Observe how the lumbar spine elongates and the belly is drawn back (softly) into the pelvic basin.

5.9I FACING WALL

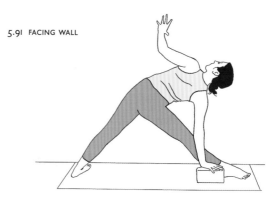

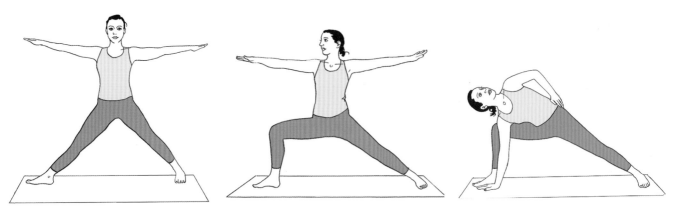

5.10A PARSVA HASTA PADASANA

5.10B BEND RIGHT LEG

5.10C RIGHT HAND ON FLOOR;
LEFT HAND ON WAIST

5.10
Utthita Parsvakonasana
Extended Side-Angle Pose

BENEFITS. Utthita Parsvakonasana builds strength in the arms and legs and improves flexibility in the hips, shoulders, and spine. Fat is reduced around the waist and hips. This pose helps the digestive and eliminatory systems to function more efficiently and also tones the internal organs and reduces the possibility of menstrual disorders.

PRACTICE. Stand on your mat in Tadasana, feet together (5.8a). Inhale and jump (or step) your feet 4 feet apart into Utthita Hasta Padasana (5.8d). Come into Parsva Hasta Padasana, by turning your right foot and leg out 90 degrees and turn your left foot slightly in (5.10a). Align your right heel with the arch of your left foot. Stretch your arms and straighten your elbows. Extend out through your fingertips and move your shoulder blades down. Lift your side ribs up and open your chest.

Keep your chest and abdomen facing forward. Exhale and bend your right leg to form a right angle (5.10b). Extend your torso sideways along your right thigh, and resting your right hand (or fingertips) on the floor and to the inside of your right foot, and your left hand on your waist (5.10c).

Press your right knee back and in line with your outer right hip and outer right ankle. Use that leverage to move your right buttock forward (5.10d, incorrect; 5.10e, correct). Press your right hand (or fingertips) into the floor, and stretch your left arm straight up (5.10f). Rotate first your pelvis and then your chest to the left. Lift and open your chest. Feel the stretch across the groins.

Fully stretch your back leg, extending through your outer left heel. (Beginners stop here.) Without disturbing your spinal rotation or allowing your front knee to roll in, switch your right hand to the outside of your right foot. Press your tailbone forward to align your pelvis over the midline.

Connect your right shoulder blade into your back, straighten your right arm and turn it out. Rotate your left arm in at the shoulder joint and stretch it diagonally over your left ear with the palm facing down. Look up (5.10g).

Press down through your left foot. Inhale and swing your left arm up and come to a standing position. Turn your feet to the front, then to the left, and repeat the pose on the other side. When you are done, jump (or step) to Tadasana.

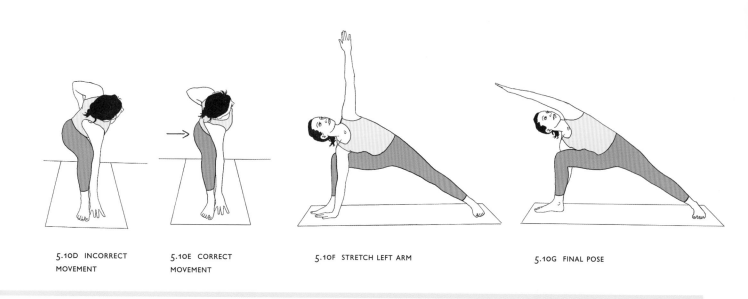

5.10D INCORRECT MOVEMENT

5.10E CORRECT MOVEMENT

5.10F STRETCH LEFT ARM

5.10G FINAL POSE

CAUTIONS. Do not practice this pose or its modifications if you have high blood pressure, if you are menstruating, or for three days following menstruation.

UTTHITA PARSVAKONASANA WITH BACK FOOT AGAINST WALL. Working with the foot braced provides a strong framework from which to properly align the pelvis and avoid straining the abdominal organs.

To begin, position the short side of your mat against the wall. Stand with your left shoulder at a right angle to the wall. Place your left hand on the wall at shoulder height. With the outer edge of your left foot against the wall, step your right foot out approximately 4 feet. With an exhalation, bend your knee to form a right angle to your shin-bone. Place your right hand on the floor, outside your right foot (5.10h).

UTTHITA PARSVAKONASANA WITH BACK AGAINST WALL. Working against the wall serves two purposes: it facilitates a greater horizontal expansion of the torso and pelvis and enables you to practice without overexerting.

Place the long end of your mat against the wall. Place a block between your right outer heel and the wall. Come into Utthita Parsvakonasana on the right and rest your right hand on the block. Roll the left side of your trunk and pelvis into the wall and away from your right, bent knee. Extend your left arm overhead. Relax your throat, eyes, and tongue, and look up (5.10i).

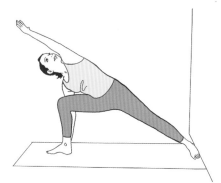

5.10H WITH BACK FOOT AGAINST WALL

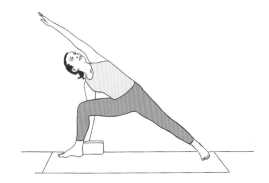

5.10I WITH BACK AGAINST WALL

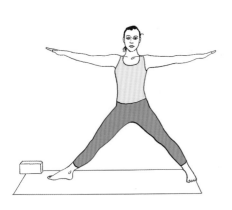

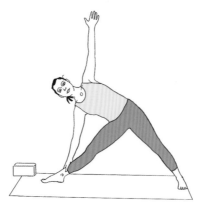

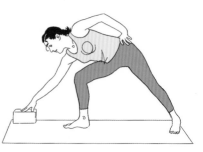

5.11A PARSVA HASTA PADASANA   5.11B UTTHITA TRIKONASANA   5.11C BEND KNEE, HAND ON BLOCK

5.11

Ardha Chandrasana
Half-Moon Pose

BENEFITS. Ardha Chandrasana is an important pose for women because it creates mobility in the hip joints and increases circulation to the abdominal organs. The front of the torso, including the lungs, is opened, which encourages the breath to flow. The posture develops balance, poise, and coordination.

PRACTICE. Place a block at one end of your mat so it is positioned about 1 foot in front of the standing leg. Stand in Tadasana (5.8a) and jump (or step) your feet 4 feet apart into Utthita Hasta Padasana (5.8d). Fully stretch your arms. Press down through your feet and lift your kneecaps. Turn your left foot in and your right foot out in Parsva Hasta Padasana (5.11a). Assume Utthita Trikonasana to the right (5.11b). Place your left hand on your waist. Step your left foot in toward your right foot, bend your right knee and, reaching out to the right side, place your right hand on the block (5.11c). Exhale and simultaneously straighten your right leg and lift your left leg (5.11d). Point your left toes forward.

Press your hand onto the block and roll your left shoulder back. Distribute your weight evenly between your right leg and right hand. Do not lean into the block. Balance your pelvis directly above your right foot, so your right leg is perpendicular to the floor. Make sure that the lifted leg is parallel to the floor and does not rise above or drop below the level of your hips.

Press down through your right leg and open your right groin by rotating your pelvis up and to the left. To avoid collapsing the lumbar spine and placing strain on the abdomen, move your right buttock bone forward.

Roll your left shoulder back and release your shoulder blades down away from your neck. Stretch your left arm up, and slowly turn your head to look at your left hand (5.11e). Extend down through your right arm and turn your right inner elbow out.

Bend your right leg and, as you exhale, carefully reach back with your left leg and return to Utthita Trikonasana. Press your outer left foot down, inhale, swing your torso to the left, and come to standing. Turn both feet forward. Move the block to the other end of the mat and repeat the pose to the left side. When done, jump (or step) your feet to Tadasana.

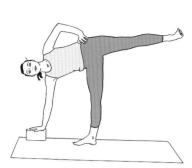

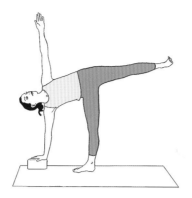

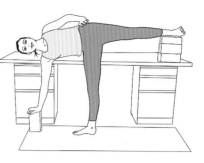

5.11D LIFT LEG

5.11E FINAL POSE

5.11F WITH LEG SUPPORT:
REST FOOT ON BOOKS

CAUTIONS. Do not practice this pose unsupported if you have knee or ankle problems or are menstruating.

ARDHA CHANDRASANA WITH LEG SUPPORT. This version can relieve lower back pain and menstrual cramps. It is beneficial for women with fibroid tumors, endometriosis, and cysts, and it helps reduce a heavy menstrual flow.

Place your mat parallel to the long side of a table. Stand on your mat, facing away from the table. A stack of books should be to your left on the table; the block should be on the mat to your right.

Come into the pose, stretching your left leg along the table, and rest your foot on the books. The books should lift your leg and foot to hip height. (You may need to experiment to get the right height.) Press your right thigh or buttock firmly against the edge of the table. Place your left hand on your hip (5.11f).

Press down through your right heel, keeping the arch of your right foot active and your inner anklebone lifted. Do not allow your belly to fall forward and away from the table. Lengthen your tailbone away from your lumbar spine. Relax the abdomen. Rotate your pelvis, chest, and left shoulder back until the chest and pelvis open to the maximum. Raise your right arm overhead and look up (5.11g).

ARDHA CHANDRASANA AGAINST WALL. If you are a beginning student, you will benefit from practicing this variation. You can practice it during

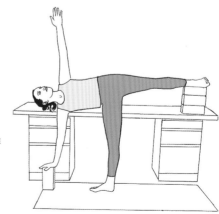

5.11G WITH LEG SUPPORT: FINAL POSE

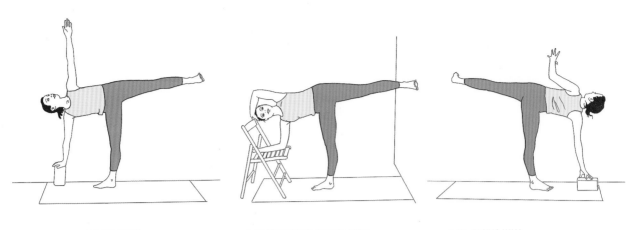

menstruation, because it does not require the same physical exertion of the other variations. It helps to reduce a heavy menstrual flow and relieves menstrual cramps. Position your mat with the long side touching the wall. Place a block at one end of the mat, about 1 foot in front of the standing leg. Once balanced in Ardha Chandrasana, exhale and roll your chest, torso, and pelvis back to the wall (5.11h).

Ardha Chandrasana with Foot Against Wall. Beginners or those who need to work in a modified way can practice with the raised foot against the wall. Depending on your flexibility, you can rest your hand on the floor, on a block, or on a chair seat. As in all modifications of Ardha Chandrasana, the raised foot should be on the same plane as your pelvis and shoulders (5.11i).

Ardha Chandrasana Facing Wall. The tendency of some women to push the belly forward can be more easily corrected when facing the wall. Ardha Chandrasana Facing Wall facilitates the proper alignment of the abdominal organs within the pelvic cavity. It reduces heaviness in the abdomen and helps alleviate congestion in the uterus. It benefits those with fibroids or any problems stemming from disease or discomfort of the pelvic organs.

Stand facing the wall with the legs 4 feet apart, turned to the right. Come into Ardha Chandrasana with your right hand on a block and your left hand on the wall. Have the toes of your left foot braced against the wall (5.11j). Revolve your left hip away from your right hip and away from the wall. Tuck your right buttock into the body to open the front of the pelvis and the right groin to the wall. This makes space for the right ovary. Draw your frontal hipbones up toward your chest and move your right back ribs toward the wall. Lift and open your chest.

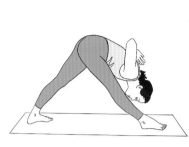

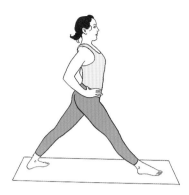

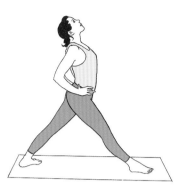

5.12A CLASSIC POSE   5.12B REVOLVE HIPS AND TORSO   5.12C RAISE CHEST, LOOK UP

5.12

Parsvottanasana
Extended Side-Stretch Pose

BENEFITS. This version of the classic pose (5.12a) strengthens the legs, releases the hamstrings, and mobilizes the hips and spine. With the hands down on either side of your front foot, you can more easily work at lengthening the lower abdomen. This is of particular benefit to women, because it helps reduce the tension and hardness around the abdominal area that can obstruct the menstrual flow or cause the flow to be heavy. It benefits those with fibroid tumors or ovarian cysts and also those whose internal reproductive organs are weak or underdeveloped, by toning and strengthening the lower abdomen.

PRACTICE. Stand on your mat in Tadasana, feet together (5.8a). With an inhalation, jump (or step) your feet approximately 3 to 3½ ft. apart into Utthita Hasta Padasana (5.8d). Extend out through your fingertips and draw your shoulder blades away from your ears. Press down through your heels and straighten your legs. Lift your chest.

Place your hands on your hips. Take Parsva Hasta Padasana (5.9a), turning your left foot in about 45 degrees to the right and turning your right foot out. Check to see that the heel of your right foot is in line with the arch of your left. Revolve your hips and torso to the right and line up the center of your chest and pelvis with the inner edge of your right leg (5.12b). Keep your legs straight and the arches of your feet active; rotate your left thigh in and back; extend down through your outer left heel; press down through the inner edge of your right foot and bring your knee cap and thigh muscle up. Spread and extend your toes from the base to the tips. Curve your spine into your back; draw your shoulder blades away from your ears. Move your tailbone in and lift your frontal hipbones. By so doing, you can avoid pushing the abdomen forward. Lift your chest and look up (5.12c).

Exhale and bend forward over your right leg. Place your hands on the floor, on either side of

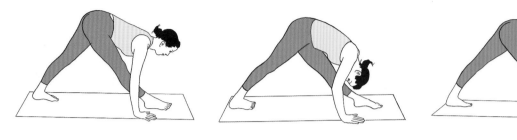

5.12D HANDS ON FLOOR   5.12E FINAL POSE   5.12F WITH BLOCKS

your right foot (5.12d). Align the pelvis to bring the abdomen parallel to the floor; press your right hip back and roll your left hip forward. Extend your chest forward and roll your shoulders back. Then, maintaining the length through both sides of the abdomen, exhale and bend forward to align your torso over your right leg (5.12e).

To change sides, place your hands on your hips and, with an inhalation, swing your trunk back to the upright position. Turn your feet first to the front, then to the left. Repeat the pose on the other side. When both sides are complete, release your hands and jump (or step) back to Tadasana.

CAUTIONS. Do not practice this pose unsupported if you have a herniated disk, a pulled hamstring, or are menstruating.

PARSVOTTANASANA WITH BLOCKS. If your hands do not reach the floor without your knees bending or your back rounding, place your hands on blocks (5.12f).

5·13
Virabhadrasana I
Warrior Pose I

BENEFITS. Virabhadrasana I, as its name suggests, will help you to develop the qualities of a warrior: physical strength and stamina, determination, focus, and bravery. The way that we hold the lower spine influences the alignment and performance of the inner organs. Through the correct practice of this pose, circulation throughout the pelvic area is boosted and a healthy functioning of the ovaries is maintained.

PRACTICE. Stand on your mat in Tadasana, feet together (5.8a). Jump (or step) your feet 4 feet apart into Parsva Hasta Padasana (5.8d). Activate the arches of your feet, spread your toes, and broaden the soles of the feet. Turn your palms to the ceiling. Raise your arms overhead and, at the same time, draw your inner thighs up (5.13a). Extend up through your fingertips and squeeze your elbows in toward each other.

Turn your torso and right foot 90 degrees and simultaneously rotate your left foot in 60 degrees. Make sure that the heel of the front foot is in line with arch of the back foot and the center of your

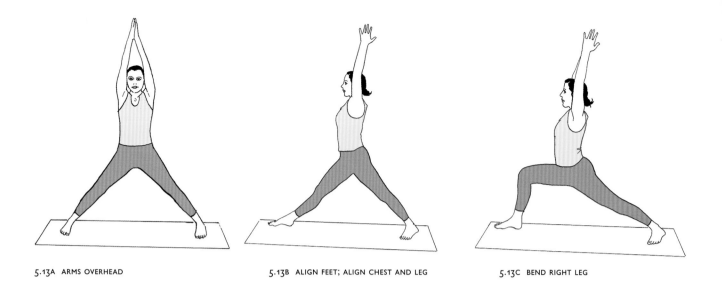

5.13A ARMS OVERHEAD   5.13B ALIGN FEET; ALIGN CHEST AND LEG   5.13C BEND RIGHT LEG

chest and pelvis lines up with the inner edge of your right leg (5.13b).

Firm your kneecaps and draw them up toward your thighs. Exhale and bend your right leg until your thigh and shin form a right angle to the floor (5.13c). Look up (5.13d).

To aid in the balanced production of hormones, blood must flow freely around the ovaries. Therefore it is imperative to not initiate this pose from the abdomen or allow the pubic bone to drop forward; these actions may compress the lumbar spine and strain the abdominal organs and constrict circulation.

Anchor the pose from your left leg, extend down and through your outer left heel, and rotate your left thigh in. Tuck the left side of your tailbone under. Move the left hipbone forward and square it with the right one. Move the perineum slightly to the front. Draw the top of the pubic bone in and up.

Align your torso so your shoulders are over your hips. Keep your hips down so your right thigh remains parallel to the floor. Press your shoulder blades into your back ribs and lift and broaden your rib cage.

Inhale and straighten your right leg. Turn your feet to the front, and repeat on the other side. When finished, jump (or step) your feet back to Tadasana.

CAUTIONS. This is one of the most strenuous of the standing poses, so do not practice it if you are menstruating or for three days following your period, or if you have bulging or herniated disks or high blood pressure.

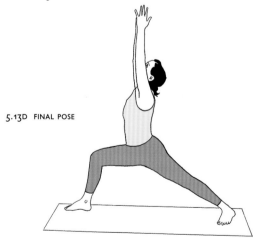

5.13D FINAL POSE

STANDING POSES AND A FLOWING SEQUENCE: BUILDING A SUPPORT SYSTEM   53

第9贴　正面　凯源-4色-WomandYoga-内页拼版.job

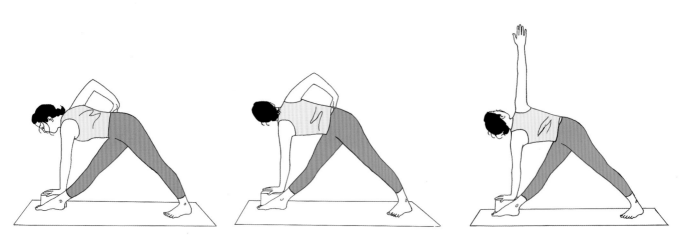

5.14A ONE HAND ON BLOCK   5.14B ROTATE TORSO   5.14C FINAL POSE

5·14

Parivrtta Trikonasana
Revolved Triangle Pose

BENEFITS. Parivrtta Trikonasana increases the circulation to the spine and keeps it healthy and flexible. It relieves lower back pain, tones the entire abdominal area, and improves balance and concentration.

PRACTICE. Stand on your mat in Tadasana, feet together (5.8a). Jump (or step) your feet 4 feet apart into Parsva Hasta Padasana (5.8d). Come into Parsvottanasana with Blocks (5.12f). Then move your left hand from the left block to the right one, and place your right hand on your hip (5.14a). With an exhalation, rotate your torso to the right. (5.14b).

Focus on the spread of the feet and on pressing down through the outer back heel. Your balance and the rotation of your torso grow from the stability of the legs.

Rather than forcing the twist from the front of the body, sink your left shoulder blade into your torso and initiate the rotation from your back ribs. Press your hand into the block and extend your torso toward your head.

Roll your right shoulder back until it is directly above your left shoulder. Stretch your right arm up and look up (5.14c). Align your head and your tailbone with the invisible line that runs between the heel of your front foot and the arch of your back foot.

Inhale and return to an upright position. Turn your feet to the front and repeat on the other side. Jump (or step) back to Tadasana.

CAUTIONS. Do not practice Parivrtta Trikonasana during menstruation, because the strong abdominal twist can irritate the uterus and disturb the menstrual process. If you have endometriosis or ovarian cysts, practice only the supported version.

PARIVRTTA TRIKONASANA WITH WALL AND CHAIR OR BLOCK. Beginners and those with fibroid tumors or scanty menstrual flow will benefit from practicing with these supported modifications, in which the abdominal area can be revolved without creating abdominal tension.

Place the short side of your mat against the wall. Place either a block or a chair at the other end, with the chair seat facing the wall. Begin with upright Parsvottanasana (5.12b), but with the heel of your left foot braced against the wall. To help stabilize the front leg, the edge of the chair

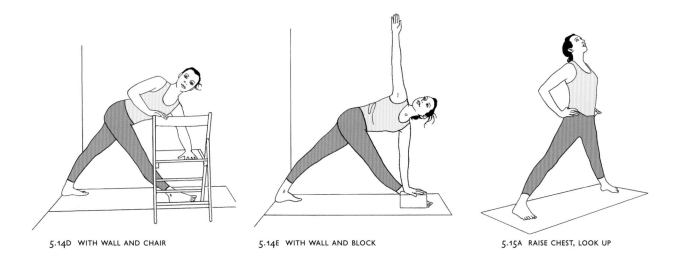

5.14D WITH WALL AND CHAIR   5.14E WITH WALL AND BLOCK   5.15A RAISE CHEST, LOOK UP

seat should press against your right outer calf. Place either your left palm on the chair seat and your right hand on the chair back (5.14d), or your left hand on the block (5.14e).

5·15
Prasarita Padottanasana
Standing Wide-Angle Pose

BENEFITS. Prasarita Padottanasana is practiced in two stages: with the head up and with the head down. Each has different benefits. When the head is up, this pose improves the circulation to and function of the ovaries and thyroid. Consequently the glandular system is brought to a healthy balance, and menstrual problems, such as irregular periods, very light or very heavy periods, or spotting between periods, are corrected.

When practiced with the head down, this pose encourages a healthy menstrual flow. It also relieves tension in the back, neck, and jaw. This stage soothes the nervous system and boosts energy. It also helps the brain recover from strain or fatigue. For beginners or those suffering from neck injuries, this stage is an alternative to Salamba Sirsasana (9.3f).

PRACTICE. Stand on your mat in Tadasana, feet together (5.8a). Place your hands on your hips. Take Utthita Hasta Padasana by jumping (or stepping) your feet 4½ to 5 feet apart (5.8d). Then place your hands back on your hips.

Hold the floor well with the soles of your feet. Spread your toes. Raise your inner anklebones and activate the arches. Lift your kneecaps and straighten your legs. Roll your shoulders back and down, raise your chest and look up (5.15a). Exhale and maintain the lift of the chest and, leading with your breastbone, bend forward from the hips (5.15b).

5.15B BEND FORWARD

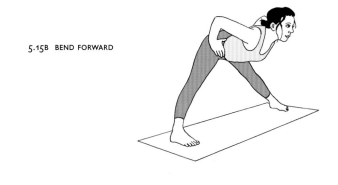

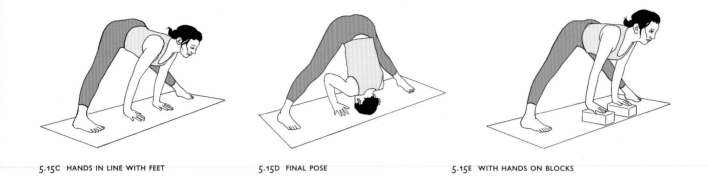

5.15C HANDS IN LINE WITH FEET   5.15D FINAL POSE   5.15E WITH HANDS ON BLOCKS

For stage one, place your hands, shoulder-width apart, on the floor and in line with your feet (5.15c). Draw your inner knees toward your inner groins and lift your sitting bones. Extend your breastbone forward and your pubic bone back. Allow maximum length to come to your spine.

Then move to the next stage: Maintaining the extension in the spine and trunk, bend your elbows back and fold your trunk forward and down. Rest the top of your head on the floor (5.15d). Your forearms should be perpendicular to the floor.

Raise your shoulders up and away from the floor and draw your shoulder blades away from your ears. Keep your elbows in line with your shoulders. Fully activate and stretch your legs and rotate your inner groins back and up. Balance toward the front of your feet and bring the legs to vertical so the hips are aligned over the feet. Allow your belly to soften and release downward.

Place your hands on your hips. Inhale and slowly swing your torso to an upright position. Move your feet slightly toward each other, and jump (or step) them together to Tadasana.

CAUTIONS. Do not practice this pose during menstruation if you are fatigued. Similarly, do not practice this or any other pose that involves bend-

ing forward if it causes dizziness (that is, if you have low blood pressure). A regular practice that includes Salamba Sirsasana (9.2d), Salamba Sarvangasana I (9.3f), Halasana (9.6d), Setu Bandha Sarvangasana (TK), and Viparita Karani (9.9d) will stabilize blood pressure levels.

In stage one, flexible women should take care not to push down heavily into the abdomen. On the other hand, those who are stiff should avoid rounding the back and sucking the abdominal organs up toward the lumbar spine by practicing Prasarita Padottanasana with Hands on Blocks (5.15e).

PRASARITA PADOTTANASANA WITH HANDS ON BLOCKS. If you are less flexible, you can practice stage one with your hands on blocks (5.15e).

PRASARITA PADOTTANASANA WITH HEAD ON BLOCK. If your head does not reach the floor in stage two, support it on a block (5.15f).

PRASARITA PADOTTANASANA WITH CHAIR AND WALL. Those with reduced mobility around the hip joints will benefit from leaning against the wall and placing the head on a chair. In addition, this modification reduces fatigue and mental strain, relaxes the abdomen, improves circulation around the ovaries and uterus, and benefits those

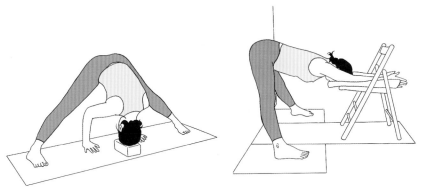

5.15F WITH HEAD ON BLOCK

5.15G WITH CHAIR AND WALL

with fibroid tumors. Practice this way during your period to relieve menstrual cramps and headaches and the tension of delayed menstruation.

Place the long side of one mat against the wall and a second mat on top of it, with the short side against the wall. Position a chair at the center the mat, with the seat facing the wall. Place a folded blanket on the seat. Stand in Tadasana (5.8a), about 1 foot from the wall, facing the chair. Step your feet 4 to 5 feet apart to Utthita Hasta Padasana (5.8d). Lean your buttocks against the wall. Place your hands on your hips and, with an exhalation, bend forward. Support your head on the chair. Thread your arms through the chair and extend them away from you, palms facing in (5.15g). Extend through your fingertips and press back through your shoulder blades. Keep your legs straight and your brain quiet. To come up, inhale and press your palms into the chair seat to push to standing. Step your feet together and come to Tadasana.

第10贴　正面 凯源-4色-WomandYoga-内页拼版.job

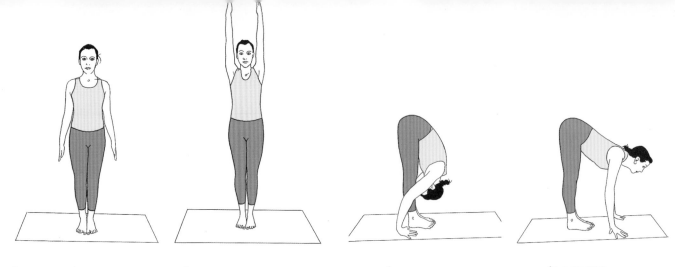

5.16A TADASANA WITH FEET TOGETHER   5.16B TADASANA URDHVA HASTASANA   5.16C UTTANASANA   5.16D RAISE HEAD

5.16

Surya Namaskara
Salute to the Sun

BENEFITS. In addition to the standing poses, this chapter includes Adho Mukha Svanasana (5.5d), Urdhva Mukha Svanasana (5.6c), Chaturanga Dandasana (5.7d) and Uttanasana (5.4c). When practiced as a continuous cycle, these postures form Surya Namaskara (5.16a through 5.16g). This particular *vinyasa*, or flowing sequence, where the emphasis is on rhythm and speed, develops alertness and stamina. It tones and cleanses the pelvic organs, strengthens the upper body, and brings the whole system to life.

PRACTICE. Start by learning each pose separately. When you are familiar with them, you are ready to put them together. Synchronize your breath with each transition, as you move from pose to pose. Take a few normal breaths in each pose before moving on to the next.

Begin in Tadasana with Feet Together (5.16a). Inhale, swing the arms up into Tadasana Urdhva Hastasana (5.16b). Exhale, swoop forward and down into Uttanasana (5.16c). Inhale; raise your head (5.16d). Exhale, jump back into Adho Mukha Svanasana (5.16e). From there, inhale as you swing forward and up into Urdhva Mukha Svanasana (5.16f); jump lightly (or pick up each foot independently) and come onto the tops of your feet. You will feel how the pelvic organs are now stretched. Exhale, bend your arms, and simultaneously hop back onto your toes and drop down into Chaturanga Dandasana (5.16g). This tones and contracts the abdominal organs. Inhale, jump lightly back onto the tops of your feet, and repeat Urdhva Mukha Svanasana (5.16f). Then exhale and, as you swing back into Adho Mukha Svanasana (5.16e), the pelvic area is flooded with a fresh blood supply. Exhale and jump forward into Uttanasana (5.16c). Inhale and, bringing your arms up with you, stand up and come to Tadasana Urdhva Hastasana. (5.16b). End in Tadasana with Feet Together (5.16a). Repeat three times.

CAUTIONS. Surya Namaskara should only be practiced *after* the menstrual and postmenstrual phases. Do not practice this or any other sequence that involves jumping if you have back or knee injuries or any other medical problem.

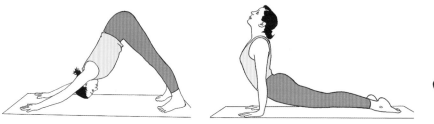

5.16E ADHO MUKHA SVANASANA

5.16F URDHVA MUKHA SVANASANA

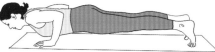

5.16G CHATTURANGA DANDASANA

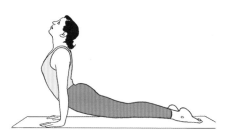

5.16F URDHVA MUKHA SVANASANA

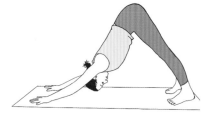

5.16E ADHO MUKHA SVANASANA

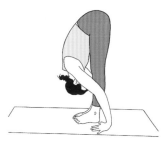

5.16C UTTANASANA

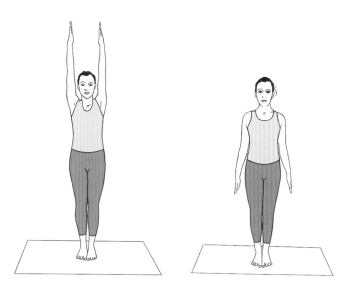

5.16B TADASANA URDHVA HASTASANA

5.16A TADASANA WITH FEET TOGETHER

6

Sitting Poses and Twists: Finding Your Center

ANY OF THE CONVENTIONS of everyday life, like sitting on chairs, working at desks, and driving cars, adversely affect the body. They cause the hips to become tight and inflexible and the knees and ankles to get stiff. In fact, too much sitting in chairs causes more stress to the spine and weaker back muscles than does standing. When you practice yoga's sitting poses and twists, you involve a wide range of motion in the pelvic, knee, and ankle joints, and flexibility rapidly improves. These poses also encourage you to use your back, and the spine is strengthened. In the early 1970s, my first yoga teacher, Penny Nield-Smith, admonished her students to throw away their chairs. Some of us did just that. (Others went to extremes and sawed the legs off their antique heirloom tables!)

Sitting poses can be especially helpful around the time of menstruation. They relieve the symptoms of premenstrual fluid retention in the legs, and when combined with forward bends they can reduce abdominal cramps, migraine headaches, low back pain, and fatigue. When combined with twists, they relieve abdominal bloating and a variety of other menstrual symptoms, including nausea and low back pain. Sitting poses also help calm and focus the mind, making it easier to draw inward and meditate.

Twists are also important for women, because they tone and strengthen the internal reproductive organs. As Geeta S. Iyengar advises in *Yoga: A Gem for Women*, menstrual disorders, malfunctioning of the endocrine glands, and obesity can all be remedied by the practice of twists. The function of the liver is also boosted with twisting poses. The liver converts potentially toxic forms of estrogen into safer forms of estrogen, and it removes metabolic waste created by the body as well as environmental toxins. Rotating the spine is like wringing out a wet towel; the stagnant blood and lymphatic fluid is squeezed out from around the abdominal area (including the liver); when the pose is released, the musculature relaxes again. Fresh blood floods into the area to bathe and renourish it. Twists also improve digestion.

General Cautions for Practicing the Sitting Poses

When practicing the sitting poses and twists presented in this chapter, remember to follow these guidelines. Cautions are also included with each pose.

■ Knees, ankles, and feet carry the weight of the body and so are important joints. Women's knees are particularly vulnerable and prone to injury. The female pelvis is wider than the male pelvis. Therefore women's thighbones tend not to hang straight from the hips, as do men's thighbones, but to fall inward, so women have more of a tendency to be knock-kneed. This misalignment places tremendous strain on the knee joint. Activities such as carrying things that are too heavy for your body weight or repetitive movement that involves impact, such as jogging (and even the weight of carrying an unborn child during pregnancy), place an additional burden on the knees and may injure them or wear away cartilage. Caution should always be taken when jumping into and out of poses, as described in chapter 5. A yoga practice that involves some *vinyasa* (a flowing sequence in which you jump from pose to pose) is energizing and beneficial, provided it is not the mainstay of your practice.

- If you have a knee injury, have had recent knee surgery, or have sore, inflamed, or swollen knees, be cautious when practicing the sitting poses and twists that involve bending the knees.

- If you experience knee pain or pressure in any of the seated poses that involve bending your knees, use appropriate support until the your knees feel comfortable. If pain persists, do not practice the pose.

- Do not attempt the revolving, side-extending, or forward-bending variations of these poses until you have mastered the upright version and are able to fully lengthen your spine.

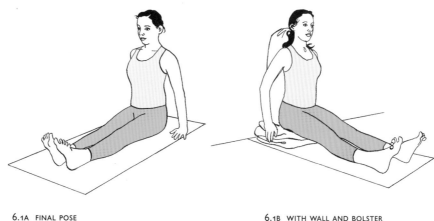

6.1A FINAL POSE

6.1B WITH WALL AND BOLSTER

6.1

Dandasana
Staff Pose

BENEFITS. Dandasana is yoga's fundamental sitting pose. It releases the hamstrings, keeps the spine strong and healthy, and tones the kidneys. You can practice Dandasana on its own or when changing from one side of a seated pose to the other. In addition, you can return to it between seated poses to straighten and rest your knees after bending them.

PRACTICE. Sit on your mat with your legs stretched out in front of you, legs and feet together. Place your fingertips on the floor and at either side of your hips (6.1a). Use your hands to draw your buttock flesh out to the sides. Without disturbing the position of the sitting bones, lean forward, take hold of your calves, and lengthen them away from you. Roll each thigh muscle in, so that both the inner and outer thighs hold the floor. Spread your toes and broaden the soles of your feet. Project the inner edges of your feet forward and draw your little toes toward you. Contact the floor with the center of each calf, thigh, and heel.

Press your fingertips and thighbones into the floor and lift your spine up. Move your sacrum in and up. Roll your shoulders back and down, and press your shoulder blades into your back. With an inhalation, lift and expand your chest. Allow the abdomen to lengthen, but do not hold it in or push it forward. Spread your collarbones out from the center.

To come out, either move on to the next sitting pose, or turn to your side and stand up.

CAUTIONS. Do not practice this pose unsupported during menstruation or if you are experiencing premenstrual tension.

DANDASANA WITH WALL AND BOLSTER. If you are menstruating or have premenstrual tension, practice this variation. Place your mat with the short end touching the wall. Sit on a folded blanket, and position an upright bolster between your back and the wall for support (6.1b).

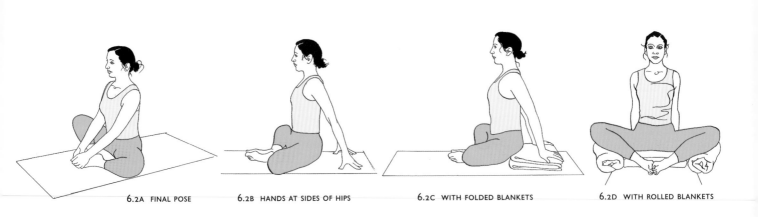

6.2A FINAL POSE   6.2B HANDS AT SIDES OF HIPS   6.2C WITH FOLDED BLANKETS   6.2D WITH ROLLED BLANKETS

6.2

Baddha Konasana
Bound-Angle Pose

BENEFITS. Baddha Konasana is an important pose for women. Stiffness in the hip joints can cause abdominal tension, which in turn can compress the pelvic organs. During menstruation, fluid retention may exacerbate this compression and cause discomfort. Baddha Konasana helps mobilize the hip joints and releases the inner thighs and groins. It tones the kidneys, exercises the abdominal organs, and relaxes the genitals. It helps to prevent leukorrhea (white vaginal discharge) and strengthens the pelvic floor, bladder, and uterus. Cystitis and pelvic inflammation are also relieved.

Patient and focused practice of Baddha Konasana stabilizes menstrual cycles marked by either heavy bleeding or a scanty flow or where there is bleeding between periods. In addition it can help to release blocked fallopian tubes.

PRACTICE. Sit on your mat in Dandasana (6.1a). Bring the soles of your feet together and let your knees fall out to the sides. Pull your feet in close to your pubic bone and hold your feet (6.2a).

If, when you sit, you allow the lumbar spine to sink down and collapse backward, then your abdomen will compress and circulation to the area will be constricted. Sit toward the front of the sitting bones, so that the front and back inner walls of the pelvis are perpendicular to the floor. Place your hands on the floor, at the sides of your hips (6.2b). Press your fingertips into the floor and, against that resistance, move your sacrum in and up. Then with an inhalation raise your side ribs. Roll your shoulders back. Lift and spread your collarbones. Extend your inner thighs toward your knees. Press your knees toward the floor. To come out, release your legs forward to Dandasana.

CAUTIONS. Do not practice this pose if you have a prolapsed or displaced uterus. If you are extremely flexible, take care not to overarch your lower back. Pushing the lumbar spine into the abdominal area may create tension in the uterus and ovaries, as well as weaken the lumbar spine. In this case, roll back onto the sitting bones and ground them. Move the sacrum back a little and lift your lower spine.

BADDHA KONASANA WITH FOLDED BLANKETS. If your knees are higher than your hips, sit on one or more folded blankets (6.2c). Having the but-

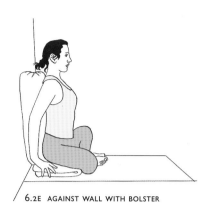

6.2E AGAINST WALL WITH BOLSTER

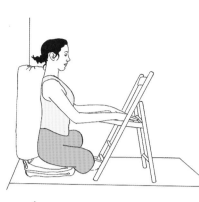

6.2F AGAINST WALL WITH CHAIR

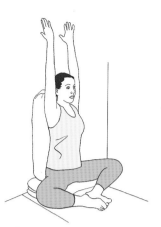

6.2G URDHVA HASTASANA
IN BADDHA KONASANA

tocks braced against the blankets provides a ful-crum from which to further release around the inner groins. It also facilitates a stronger lift of the spine. Slide forward off the blankets, until your buttocks are barely touching the floor.

BADDHA KONASANA WITH ROLLED BLANKETS. If you feel tension in your hips, or a pulling sensation at your inner thighs, or pain in the knees while practicing Baddha Konasana, place a rolled blanket under each bent knee (6.2d). When the message of support is received by the outer thighs, your impulse to grip around the hip joints dissolves, and the thighs release in their sockets. To facilitate a greater lift through the pelvis, place your hands on blocks placed at your sides.

BADDHA KONASANA AGAINST WALL WITH BOLSTER. This variation can be practiced during menstruation or if you are suffering from premenstrual tension. Sit on one or more folded blankets, placed against the wall (6.2e). Support your back against a bolster that is placed vertically against the wall.

BADDHA KONASANA AGAINST WALL WITH CHAIR OR BLOCKS. Set up as for Baddha Konasana Against Wall with Bolster (6.2e), and rest your hands on a chair seat (or beside you on blocks), so you have more leverage with which to lift the spine (6.2f).

URDHVA HASTASANA IN BADDHA KONASANA. This variation strengthens and creates space around the uterus, ovaries, and fallopian tubes. It helps to keep the shoulder joints flexible and the arms strong.

Sit on two folded blankets placed near a wall, in Baddha Konasana. Support your back against a vertical bolster. With your palms facing each other, inhale and swing your arms forward and then up overhead (6.2g). Extend through your fingers and straighten your elbows. Press your shoulder blades into your back. Align your arms alongside your ears. Against the resistance of the strong upward lift of the arms, release the muscles around your shoulder blades away from your ears.

URDHVA BADDHANGULLYASANA IN BADDHA KONASANA. This variation lengthens the spine and creates space around the uterus, ovaries, and fallopian tubes. It also helps to keep the shoulder, elbow, and wrist joints flexible and improves circulation to the breasts.

Sit on two folded blankets placed against a wall, in Baddha Konasana. Support your back against an upright bolster. Interlace your fingers. Turn your palms out and stretch your arms forward. Roll your shoulders back and down. Inhale and stretch your arms overhead alongside your

第12贴　正面　凯源-4色-WomandYoga-内页拼版.job

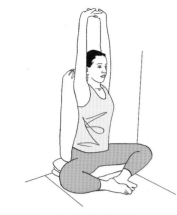

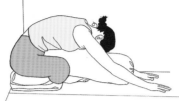

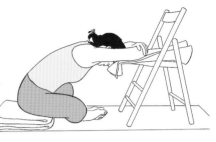

6.2H URDHVA BADDHANGULLYASANA
IN BADDHA KONASANA

6.2I ADHO MUKHA BADDHA KONASANA
WITH WALL AND BOLSTER

6.2J ADHO MUKHA BADDHA KONASANA
WITH CHAIR

ears. Extend up through the inner elbows to the inner wrists and the knuckles of the index fingers (6.2h). To change sides, bring your arms back, level with your shoulders. Turn your palms toward you. Change the interlock so the opposite thumb is on top, and repeat the pose.

ADHO MUKHA BADDHA KONASANA WITH WALL AND BOLSTER. This variation relieves lower back pain and fatigue, soothes the nerves, and calms the brain. It dramatically increases the flexibility and circulation in the hip joints. Sit on your mat on two folded blankets placed against the wall. Put a bolster lengthwise on top of your feet, with the end touching your abdomen. Wiggle your sitting bones back, to where the floor and the wall meet. With an exhalation, extend your torso forward, lengthening the front of your spine from the navel to the throat. Rest your torso and forehead on the bolster (6.2i). If you need more height, place a folded blanket under your forehead.

ADHO MUKHA BADDHA KONASANA WITH CHAIR. Here is an even gentler way of practicing Adho Mukha Baddha Konasana that may help reduce a heavy flow during menstruation. Fold your arms and rest your head on a chair seat (6.2j). Those with fibroid tumors or uterine cysts (as well as those with restricted movement around the hips

and pelvis) will also benefit, as the abdominal organs are less likely to be restricted. Use some padding under your head and feet if necessary for comfort.

ADHO MUKHA BADDHA KONASANA WITH BLOCK. Do not go forward in this pose if your knees are higher than your hips in Baddha Konasana. If you are flexible, you can practice Adho Mukha Baddha Konasana by placing your forehead on a block (or on the floor) (6.2k).

LEANING BADDHA KONASANA. This pose creates space around the pelvic organs and torso and increases circulation to the abdominal organs, including the uterus and liver. Abdominal tension is reduced and menstrual cramping associated with endometriosis is relieved. It benefits women who experience extreme nausea around menstruation, as well as those suffering from diarrhea, irritable bowel syndrome, and acid reflux.

Place the short side of your mat against the wall. Position a chair with its back against the wall. Place a second mat, folded into four, on the chair seat, and a folded blanket at the foot of the chair. Position two blocks, side by side, on the chair seat. Place two folded blankets on top of the blocks. Adjust the blankets according to your height and flexibility and according to where you

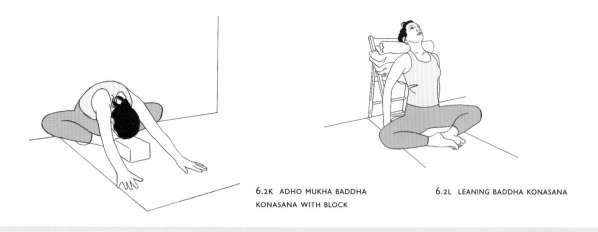

6.2K ADHO MUKHA BADDHA
KONASANA WITH BLOCK

6.2L LEANING BADDHA KONASANA

get the most extension, relief, and support when you are in the pose. Have a rolled blanket ready to support your neck.

Sit in front of the chair on the blanket. Bring the soles of your feet together. Lean back and over the blankets. Place the blanket roll behind your neck, so your throat stretches and your forehead slopes back. Take care that your head is sufficiently supported and does not roll to the side. Place your hands on the floor beside you. (6.2l)

Roll your shoulders back and slide them away from your ears. Against the resistance of your fingers and thumbs pressing into the floor, pull your trunk and chest up. Press your thighs to the floor. Feel the resulting opening at the hip joints and the lengthening and stretching of the abdomen and chest. Relax your eyes and tongue. Allow your head to become cool and rested.

To come out, sit upright. Bend your knees and turn over onto your right side. Rest here before standing.

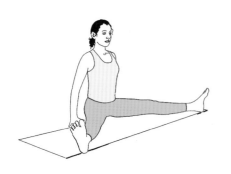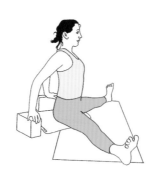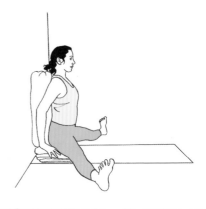

6.3A FINAL POSE   6.3B WITH BLANKET AND BLOCKS   6.3C WITH WALL AND BOLSTER

6.3

Upavistha Konasana
Seated Wide-Angle Pose

BENEFITS. This pose is particularly beneficial for women. It increases the circulation to the lower abdomen, widens and relaxes the pelvic floor, and reduces any obstruction to the menstrual flow. In addition, those with blocked fallopian tubes, irritation or burning sensations around the genital organs, leukorrhea (white vaginal discharge), pelvic inflammation, ovarian cysts, endometriosis, or any menstrual disorders benefit from its practice.

PRACTICE. Sit on your mat in Dandasana (6.1a). Separate your legs and stretch them out toward your heels. Place your hands on the floor beside your hips. Press your fingers into the floor, raise your pelvis up off the floor, and slide it forward, without disturbing the feet, to widen the legs a little more. Sit back down on the center of your sitting bones. Press your thighs and shinbones into the floor. Inhale and lift your torso and chest up (6.3a). Maintain the lift of the chest as you exhale.

Move your sacrum in and up. Release the

shoulder blades down and coil them into your back to help support and open the chest more. Roll your thighs in slightly and position your heels at the center, so that the feet remain upright, not rolled out. Flex your toes. To come out, slide your legs back to Dandasana.

CAUTIONS. If you are extremely flexible, take care not to overarch your lower back. Pushing the lumbar into the abdominal area can create tension in the uterus and ovaries, as well as weaken the lumbar spine. In this case, roll back onto the sitting bones and ground them. Move the sacrum back a little and lift your lower spine.

UPAVISTHA KONASANA WITH BLANKET AND BLOCKS. If you find it difficult to sit up straight with your chest expanded and your knees straight, sit on the corner of one or more folded blankets and place your hands behind you on blocks (6.3b). Lean back onto your hands, and draw your spinal column into your back. As you practice and gain flexibility in your hips and hamstrings, gradually move forward into an upright position

UPAVISTHA KONASANA WITH WALL AND BOLSTER. During menstruation, support yourself with a vertical bolster placed against the wall (6.3c).

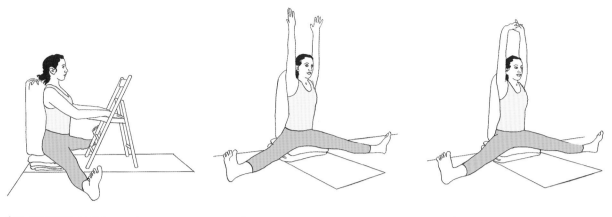

6.3D WITH WALL, BOLSTER, AND CHAIR

6.3E URDHVA HASTASANA IN UPAVISTHA KONASANA

6.3F URDHVA BADDHANGULLYASANA IN UPAVISTHA KONASANA

UPAVISTHA KONASANA WITH WALL, BOLSTER, AND CHAIR. During menstruation, support your torso with a bolster placed against the wall and rest your forearms on a chair to lessen the effort of keeping the spine straight and the chest lifted (6.3d).

URDHVA HASTASANA IN UPAVISTHA KONASANA. Raising the arms over the head brings the pelvic organs into alignment and boosts the circulation around the ovaries and uterus. It also strengthens the back and relieves stiffness in the shoulders.

Sit on your mat against the wall, on two folded blankets, in Upavistha Konasana. Support your torso with a vertical bolster. With your palms facing each other, inhale and swing them forward and up over your head (6.3e). Stretch up through your fingers and squeeze your elbows in. Press your shoulder blades into your back. Against the resistance of your extended arms, release the muscles around your shoulder blades away from your ears. Make sure your arms remain in line with your ears. Experience the stretch along both sides of your torso.

URDHVA BADDHANGULLYASANA IN UPAVISTHA KONASANA. Sit on your mat against the wall, on two folded blankets, in Upavistha Konasana. Support your torso with a vertical bolster. Interlock

your hands. Turn your palms out and extend your arms out in front of you, level with your shoulder. Straighten your arms by squeezing your inner elbows toward each other and draw your upper arms back into your shoulder joints. Stretch your arms over your head and turn the palms to face the ceiling (6.3f). Lower your arms to shoulder level and then drop them down to your sides.

LEANING UPAVISTHA KONASANA. This pose is a continuation of Leaning Baddha Konasana and has similar benefits, with the addition of increased horizontal extension of the pelvic floor and lower abdomen. Set up as for Leaning Baddha Konasana (6.2l) and then spread your legs wide apart (6.3g).

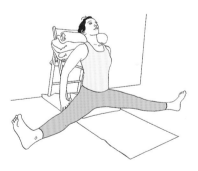

6.3G LEANING UPAVISTHA KONASANA

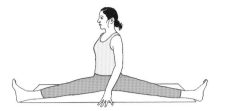

6.4A TURN TORSO TO RIGHT

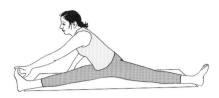

6.4B HOLD OUTSIDE OF RIGHT FOOT

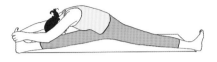

6.4C FINAL POSE

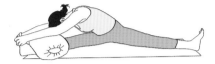

6.4D WITH BOLSTER

6.4

Parsva Upavistha Konasana
Seated Wide-Angle Sidebend Pose

BENEFITS. In addition to the benefits described for Upavistha Konasana (6.3a), this pose relieves lower back pain and increases mobility in the spine.

PRACTICE. This pose is practiced in two stages. Begin in Upavistha Konasana (6.3a). Press your fingertips on the floor, to either side of your right thigh, and turn your torso to face your right foot (6.4a). Extend back through your left inner heel and press your left thigh to the floor. Draw your sacrum in and up, and raise your side ribs. Roll your shoulders back and down.

With an exhalation, reach forward and catch the outside of your right foot with your left hand (6.4b). Press the fingertips of your right hand into the floor; draw your sacrum in, and extend your right side ribs toward your left foot. Curve your spine in and up and raise your chest. Look up.

For stage two, bring your head down. Initiating the side-bend not from the spine but from the side ribs, extend your torso along your right thigh. Clasp your right foot with both hands. Rest your

forehead on your shinbone. Roll your navel to the right. Move your shoulders away from your neck. After you have caught hold of your foot with both hands, bend your elbows out to the sides and raise them. If you are flexible, turn your hands out and clasp your left wrist with your right hand (6.4c).

If it is difficult for you to release into this pose due to tension or tight hamstrings, change sides frequently to keep a dynamic energy flowing through your spine. To come out, inhale and return to an upright position. Turn to the front and repeat the pose to the opposite side. When done, return to Dandasana.

CAUTIONS. Do not practice this pose or its variations if you have herniated or bulging disks. Do not practice this pose until you are able to sit upright with straight legs in Upavistha Konasana.

PARSVA UPAVISTHA KONASANA WITH BOLSTER. The emphasis during menstruation is to relax. Always support your head when practicing at this time, to facilitate abdominal release, calm nerves, and quiet breathing. Sit on the corner of a folded blanket. Place a bolster across your thighs to support your head (6.4d).

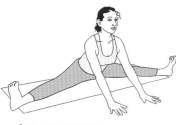

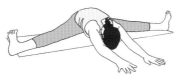

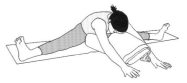

6.5A BEND FORWARD 6.5B FINAL POSE 6.5C WITH BOLSTER AND BLANKET

6.5
Adho Mukha Upavistha Konasana
Seated Wide-Angle Pose with Forward Bend

BENEFITS. Adho Mukha Upavistha Konasana is a wonderful asana for women. The sacral area is moved into a concave position, which reduces compression and heaviness in the abdomen and causes the blood to circulate properly around the pelvic area. It stimulates the ovaries and controls and regularizes the menstrual flow. Additionally it calms the nerves and helps reduce migraine headaches.

PRACTICE. This pose is practiced in two stages. To begin, sit on your mat in Upavistha Konasana (6.3a). With an exhalation, bend forward from your hips and place your hands a few feet in front of you on the floor (6.5a). Press your thighs and the tops of your shinbones to the floor. Extend through the soles of your feet. Roll your sacrum in and curve your spine forward and up. With an inhalation, lift and open your chest. Look up. If you are menstruating, pass briefly through this stage before taking your head down.

When you have achieved a strong upward lift of the spine, you can continue with stage two, which is the full forward bend. With an exhalation and leading with your breastbone, place your head, or if possible your chin, on the floor (6.5b). With each exhalation, extend your torso and chest farther forward. Keep your sit bones grounded. Breathe evenly and steadily. To come out, keep the spine curved in and the head lifted and sit up. Bring your legs back to Dandasana.

CAUTIONS. If you feel pain along the ligaments of your inner knees, draw them a little closer together. Women sometimes experience an inflammation of the ligaments around the sacroiliac joint, especially during menstruation. If this is the case, do not push yourself into a deep forward bend.

ADHO MUKHA UPAVISTHA KONASANA WITH BOLSTER AND BLANKET. Sit on the corner of a folded blanket in Upavistha Konasana (6.3a). Place a bolster, lengthwise, in front of you, with the near end close to your pelvis. Position a folded blanket at the far end. Move very gently forward over the bolster, so your abdomen and chest are supported. Rest your forehead on the blanket. Stretch your arms out in front of you (6.5c). Allow your

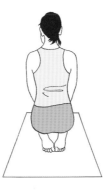

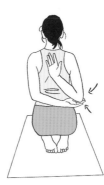

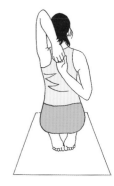

6.6A BEGIN IN VAJRASANA

6.6B GUIDE RIGHT HAND WITH LEFT HAND

6.6C FINAL POSE

brain to rest and quietness to penetrate your whole body.

ADHO MUKHA UPAVISTHA KONASANA WITH CHAIR. If you are suffering from a migraine headache or nausea, or if you have limited mobility around the pelvis and hip joints, rest your forehead and arms on a chair (6.5d).

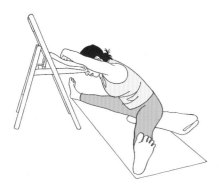

6.5D WITH CHAIR

6.6

Gomukhasana in Vajrasana
Kneeling Cow Face Pose

BENEFITS. This pose creates flexibility in the shoulder joints and upper spine. Geeta Iyengar suggests that women take the opportunity to work on the shoulders during menstruation, since the more active poses cannot be practiced at this time. (The same applies to the next pose, Paschima Namaskarasana in Vajrasana.)

PRACTICE. Sit on your mat, on your heels with your feet together (6.6a). Place your palms on your thighs. Allow the weight of your thighs to stretch the front of the ankle joints. Sit up straight and lift your chest. Extend your right arm out to the side, and then bend it behind your back. Slide the back of your hand up your back between your shoulder blades, with the fingers pointing up. Use

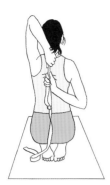

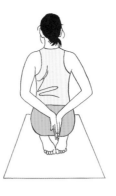

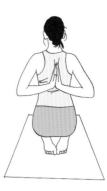

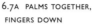

6.7A PALMS TOGETHER,
FINGERS DOWN

6.7B FINAL POSE

your left hand to guide your right hand farther up (6.6b). Raise your left arm. Bend at the elbow and drop your left hand down to meet your right. Clasp your fingers together (6.6c).

Move your left forearm in, close to your head. Roll your right shoulder back and open your right collarbone. Press your shoulder blades into your back. Lift and open your chest. Breathe evenly. Release the grip of the hands. Stretch the left arm up and sweep it out to the sides and down. Slide the right arm down. Repeat on the other side. To come out, release the grip of the hands. Sweep the right arm out to the side and down. Slide the left arm down.

CAUTION. Do not practice this pose if you have a cardiac condition.

GOMUKHASANA IN VAJRASANA WITH STRAP. If you cannot clasp your fingers, use a strap to hold the hands in place behind your back (6.6d).

6.7

Paschima Namaskarasana in Vajrasana
Kneeling Prayer Pose

BENEFITS. Paschima Namaskarasana creates freedom in the shoulders, elbows, and wrists, and promotes flexibility in the upper back.

PRACTICE. Sit on your mat, on your heels and with your feet together (6.6a). Sit up straight and open your chest. Encircle your arms behind your back and bring the palms together, fingers facing down (6.7a). Turn your hands in and up.

Slide your hands as far up the back as possible (6.7b). Press the palms together. Focus on pressing the knuckles of the index fingers and the thumbs together. Roll your shoulders back, move your upper arms toward the back of your shoulder joint, and open your collarbones. Lift and open your chest. To come out, slide your hands down.

CAUTION. Do not practice this asana if you have a cardiac condition.

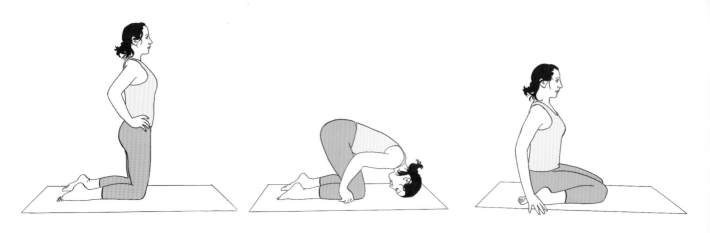

6.8A KNEELING POSITION   6.8B EASE CALF MUSCLES OUT   6.8C FINAL POSE

6.8

Virasana
Hero's Pose

BENEFITS. Virasana improves blood circulation to the knees and ankles and enhances their mobility. It reduces stiffness in the hips and relieves tired and achy legs.

PRACTICE. To begin, sit on your mat in Dandasana (6.1a). Fold your legs under you and come into a kneeling position (6.8a). Place your feet approximately 12 inches apart. Before settling into the pose, take some time to create space in the back of the knee joints. With your thumbs, ease your calf muscles out and away from the backs of your knees (6.8b). Check that your feet are pointing straight back in line with the center of your shins. Settle back down and sit between your feet. With your hands, draw your inner heels away from your inner ankles. Place your hands on the floor by the side of your hips. Sit erect (6.8c).

Ground your sitting bones and allow the tops of your thighs to descend. Press your fingers and thumbs into the floor. Against that resistance, lift your torso and spine up. Roll your shoulders back and release your shoulder blades away from your ears. Open your chest and spread your collarbones.

To come out, swivel your legs to the side and then out in front of you. Sit in Dandasana. Hold the back of each thigh individually, with your fingers interlaced, and stretch out the back of each leg.

CAUTIONS. If you have a knee injury or if you are recovering from knee surgery, work with the guidance of an experienced yoga teacher. If you experience pain or pressure in your knees while practicing this pose, come out immediately and practice Virasana with Block or Blanket for Knee Pain instead (6.8d).

VIRASANA WITH BLOCK OR BLANKET FOR KNEE PAIN. Do not force in order to sit on the floor between your shins. Sit on a block (6.8d). If you still experience discomfort in your knees, place one or more folded blankets between the backs of your thighs and your calves (6.8e). Place the blanket to within an inch of the back of the knee joints.

VIRASANA WITH BLANKET FOR STIFF ANKLES. If your ankle joints are stiff, place a lengthwise-folded blanket under your ankles, so that your toes fall off behind the blanket (6.8f).

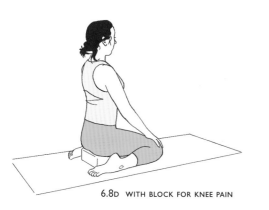

6.8D WITH BLOCK FOR KNEE PAIN

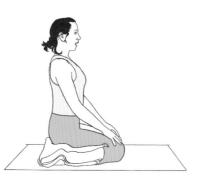

6.8E WITH BLANKET FOR KNEE PAIN

URDHVA BADDANGULLYASANA IN VIRASANA. Raising the arms with the hands interlocked helps to reduce premenstrual heaviness and relieve soreness in the breasts. This pose tones the internal organs, strengthens the arms, and mobilizes the shoulder joints.

Sit on your mat in Virasana (6.8c). Interlace your fingers, turn your palms out, and stretch your arms out in front of you. Roll your shoulders back, away from your wrists. Inhale and raise your arms over your head and in line with your ears. Squeeze your outer, upper arms toward each other, and extend up through your inner elbows into the wrists and the knuckles of your index fingers (6.8g). Allow your torso to lengthen as you press your hands up. Take care not to push your lumbar spine forward.

To change sides, lower your arms so your hands are level with your shoulders. Turn your palms toward you. Change the interlock of your fingers and repeat. To come out, lower your arms until they are level with your head. Release the interlock and return your palms to your thighs.

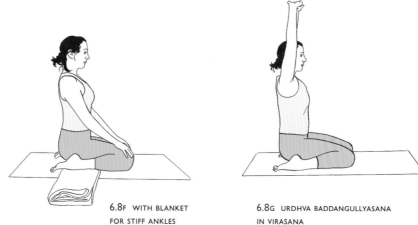

6.8F WITH BLANKET
FOR STIFF ANKLES

6.8G URDHVA BADDANGULLYASANA
IN VIRASANA

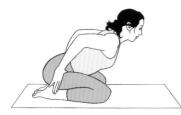

6.9A THUMBS IN HIP CREASES

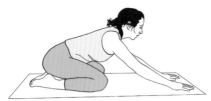

6.9B FOLD FORWARD

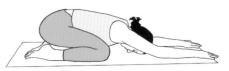

6.9C FINAL POSE

6.9

Adho Mukha Virasana
Downward-Facing Hero's Pose

BENEFITS. Adho Mukha Virasana has many of the benefits of the seated forward bends in which the nerves are soothed and the brain rested. Additionally those with tight hamstrings can practice this pose without the struggle that is sometimes experienced in many of the other forward bends.

Adho Mukha Virasana relaxes the muscles of the lower back. Practice it to relieve the lumbar spine after Supta Virasana (8.4c). This pose also helps relieve constipation, abdominal bloating and flatulence, and high blood pressure. Practice it following Salamba Sirsasana (9.2d), to release the back of the neck and to cool the body and brain.

PRACTICE. Sit on your mat in Virasana (6.8a). Bring your toes together and your knees apart. Tuck your thumbs into your hip creases (6.9a). Exhaling, fold your torso forward between your thighs (6.9b). Stretch your arms out in front of you. Press your hands, particularly the mounds of the index fingers, into the floor. Rest your forehead on the floor (6.9c). Allow your buttocks to drop toward

your heels and extend your chest toward your hands. As your head touches the floor, relax your eyes inward. To come out, sit up and swivel your legs out to the side and then out in front of you. Sit in Dandasana.

CAUTIONS. Avoid this pose if you have diarrhea or bronchitis.

ADHO MUKHA VIRSASANA WITH FOLDED BLANKET. If you feel any discomfort in your knees or if they are stiff, place a folded blanket between your thighs and calves (6.9d).

ADHO MUKHA VIRASANA WITH BOLSTER. This variation is particularly restful around the time of menstruation. It alleviates anxiety, migraine headache and for some, it eases menstrual cramps.

Place a bolster across the top of your mat. Fold forward and rest your forehead on the bolster. Extend your arms out in front of you, palms facing in, and place your forearms on the bolster (6.9e). Keep your buttocks close to your ankles. Allow the stretch of the arms to open the shoulder joints and rib cage. Fully extend your hands and fingers.

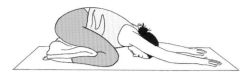

6.9D WITH FOLDED BLANKET

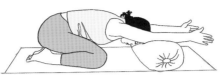

6.9E WITH BOLSTER

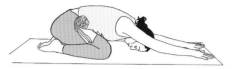

6.9F WITH BLANKET ROLL

ADHO MUKHA VIRASANA WITH BLANKET ROLL. This variation helps relieve low back pain. Place a rolled blanket across the very tops of your thighs. Fold forward over the roll and stretch your arms out in front of you. Rest your head on the floor (6.9f), or support it on a block or folded blanket.

6.10

Parsva Virasana
Hero's Pose to the Side

BENEFITS. Parsva Virasana relieves premenstrual lower back pain and, for some, abdominal cramps. Abdominal bloating is reduced.

PRACTICE. Place a block on your mat, so it is behind you when you sit in Virasana (6.8c). If your feel any knee discomfort, sit in Virasana with Block or Blanket for Knee Pain (6.8d and 6.8e).

Place your right hand behind you and on the block, and the back of your left hand against the outside of your right leg. Maintaining an upright spine, exhale and turn to the right (6.10a).

Move your shoulder blades away from your neck and press your right shoulder blade into your back. Lift your chest and spread your collarbones. Roll your right shoulder back and, syn-

chronizing with the breath (inhale and lift, exhale and turn), continue to rotate your torso to the right around the central axis of the body. Feel the weight evenly on your sitting bones. Feel your waist getting thinner and your upper chest getting broader, as you spiral upward. To work through any stiffness in the spine and torso, you can do this pose as many as 4 to 6 times on each side, moving more deeply into the pose with each repetition.

Come back to Virasana. Repeat on the left side. To come out, sit off your feet and swing your legs out in front of you in Dandasana.

CAUTION. If you are a beginning student, you can sit in Vajrasana instead (6.6a).

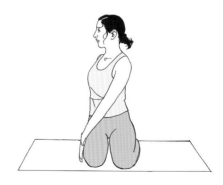

6.10A FINAL POSE

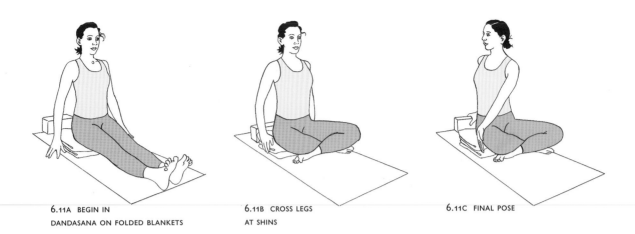

6.11A BEGIN IN
DANDASANA ON FOLDED BLANKETS

6.11B CROSS LEGS
AT SHINS

6.11C FINAL POSE

6.11

Parsva Swastikasana
Simple Cross-Leg Pose to the Side

BENEFITS. The benefits of this pose are similar to those of Parsva Virasana (6.10a). In Parsva Swastikasana, it is easier to roll the sacrum in, lift the torso, and twist. In addition, this pose removes stiffness in the hips.

PRACTICE. Place a block on your mat so it is behind you. Sit on your mat in Dandasana, place one or more folded blankets under your sitting bones to lift your lower back up out of the pelvis and release the hip sockets (6.11a).

Come into Swastikasana by crossing your legs at the shins (6.11b). Draw your heels toward your torso, and allow your knees to fall out to the sides. Sit up straight. Place the back of your left hand against your outer right thigh. Swing your right hand behind you and place your hand on the block. Inhale and lift. Exhale and revolve your torso to the right (6.11c). Hold your head directly in line with your tailbone. Continue raising your side ribs. Release your shoulder blades away from your ears and press into your back. Roll your left shoulder back. Spread your collarbones out from the center. Return to face the front. Change the cross of your legs and repeat the rotation to the left. To come out, release your legs forward into Dandasana.

CAUTION. Do not attempt to rotate your spine until you are able to fully lift the torso, with the sacrum moving in toward the pubic bone.

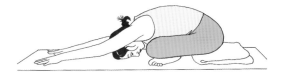

6.12A FINAL POSE

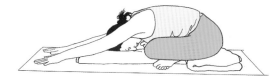

6.12B WITH BLANKET   6.12C WITH BLOCK

6.12

Adho Mukha Swastikasana
Downward-Facing Cross-Leg Pose

BENEFITS. Adho Mukha Swastikasana reduces stiffness in the hips and massages and energizes the abdominal organs. It is particularly restful during menstruation. It reduces lower back pain, removes fatigue, relieves migraine headaches, and calms the mind.

PRACTICE. Sit on your mat in Swastikasana (6.11b). Fold forward. Stretch your arms out in front of you and place your hands on the floor. Keeping your sitting bones firmly grounded, walk your hands out even more and place your head on the floor (6.12a). Elongate your front ribs away from your pelvis. Allow the skin over your front ribs to extend toward your outstretched hands and the skin on your back ribs to descend toward the floor. Breathe evenly. To come out, raise your torso and sit in Swastikasana.

CAUTIONS. Do not practice this pose if you have herniated disks or other back problems.

ADHO MUKHA SWASTIKASANA WITH BLANKET. If your outer ankle bones press uncomfortably into the floor, place a lengthwise-folded blanket under them (6.12b).

ADHO MUKHA SWASTIKASANA WITH BLOCK. If your head does not touch the floor easily, support it on a block (6.12c).

ADHO MUKHA SWASTIKASANA WITH CHAIR. If you are suffering from nausea or migraine, you can support your head on a chair (6.12d).

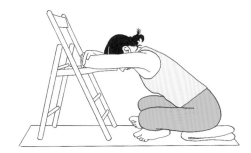

6.12D WITH CHAIR

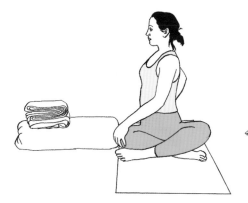

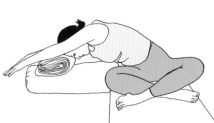

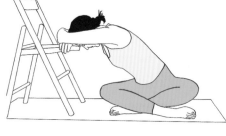

6.13A PARSVA SWASTIKASANA

6.13B FINAL POSE WITH BOLSTER AND BLANKET

6.13C FINAL POSE WITH CHAIR

6.13

Parsva Adho Mukha Swastikasana
Side-Bending Simple Cross-Leg Pose

BENEFITS. Parsva Adho Mukha Swastikasana is helpful during both the premenstrual and active bleeding phases of the cycle because it relieves low back pain, abdominal bloating, and, for some, menstrual cramps. It also reduces high blood pressure and reduces a low fever.

PRACTICE. Place a bolster or a chair facing inward at right angles to your mat. Position a folded blanket at the far end of the bolster. Assume Parsva Swastikasana to the right (6.13a). Exhale and fold down to the right so your trunk almost forms a right angle to your pelvis. Rest your head and arms on the bolster and blanket (6.13b) or, if you are less flexible, on the chair seat (6.13c).

Come out the way that you went in: sit up and return to Parsva Swastikasana. Face forward and sit in Swastikasana. Move the bolster or chair to the other side and turn to the left. Change your cross legs and repeat on the other side. Release your legs forward and sit in Dandasana (6.1a).

CAUTION. Do not practice this pose if you have knee problems.

PARSVA ADHO MUKHA SWASTIKASANA WITH HEAD TO SIDE. To relieve migraine headache, practice this side bend with your head turned to the side. Place a folded blanket on the chair seat for comfort. Hold the sides of the chair. Turn your head to the right and place the left side of your head and your left ear on the seat (6.13d). To practice to the other side, sit up, reverse the cross of your legs, and rest the right side of your head on the chair seat.

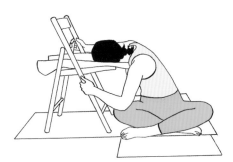

6.13D FINAL POSE WITH HEAD TO SIDE

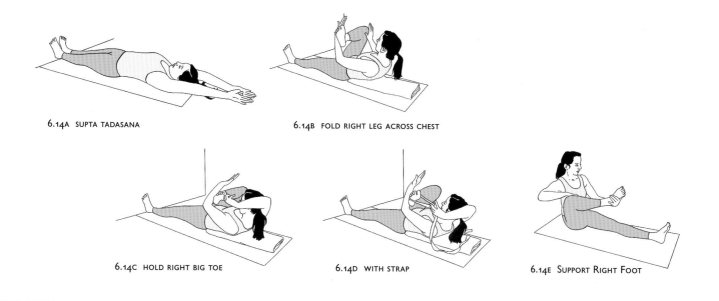

6.14A SUPTA TADASANA

6.14B FOLD RIGHT LEG ACROSS CHEST

6.14C HOLD RIGHT BIG TOE

6.14D WITH STRAP

6.14E SUPPORT RIGHT FOOT

6.14

Padmasana
Lotus Pose

BENEFITS. Padmasana is such an important pose for women that, despite the difficulties of learning it without the help of a teacher, it is included here. It tones the abdomen, strengthens the spine, and creates flexibility in the hips, knees, and ankles.

Padmasana is particularly beneficial for women when combined with reclining poses and inverted postures, although the latter combination is beyond the scope of this book. These pose combinations increase circulation to the abdominal organs and are helpful for women suffering from fibroid tumors and ovarian cysts. Padmasana can be practiced during menstruation, but only if it can be achieved without difficulty and with a minimum of preparation.

WARM-UP: SUPTA PADANGUSTHASANA III. Start by preparing your hip joints. To begin, follow the instructions for Supta Padangustasana I and II (see chapter 8).

Then, still lying on the floor, continue with Supta Padangusthasana III. Lie on your mat in Supta Tadasana (6.14a). Fold your right leg across your chest (6.14b). Raise your head and upper back off the floor. Support your right ankle in your left elbow and draw your foot toward you. With your right hand, gently direct your right knee away from you, so your knee and ankle are the same distance from your head. Raise your foot to the level of your knee. Check that both shoulders are equidistant from the floor. Line up the center of your shinbone with the center of your breastbone. Circle your right hand behind your head, rest your head in the crook of your elbow, and take hold of your right big toe with your right hand (6.14c). If you cannot reach your foot, practice with a strap (6.14d).

Externally revolve your right thigh at the hip socket. Extend from your inner right groin to your inner right knee. Roll your outer right hip away from you. Press your left thigh to the floor. With an exhalation, extend out through your inner left foot and spread your toes. Repeat on the other side.

PRACTICE. If you can do these preparations with ease and without knee pain, then you are ready to move into Padmasana. Sit on your mat in Dandasana (6.1a). Raise your right shin and support your right foot with your left hand (6.14e). Place your right foot on top of your left thigh, with the

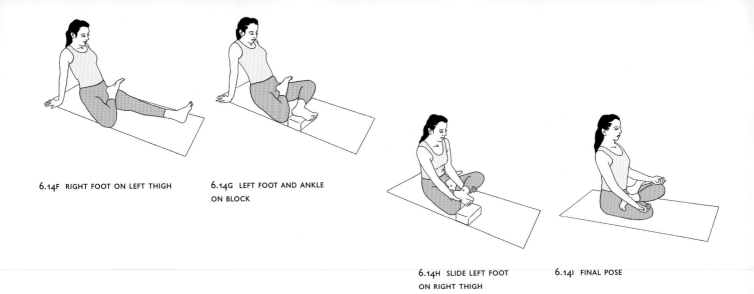

6.14F RIGHT FOOT ON LEFT THIGH

6.14G LEFT FOOT AND ANKLE
ON BLOCK

6.14H SLIDE LEFT FOOT
ON RIGHT THIGH

6.14I FINAL POSE

sole of your foot facing the ceiling (6.14f). Lean back on your hands. Use your right hip muscles to extend out through your inner right knee and slowly pump your right knee up and down a few times to the floor.

Place a block in front of your right knee. Bend your left knee and place your left foot and ankle on the block (6.14g). If your right knee can be pressed to the floor, you can proceed with Padmasana. Allow your left hip joint to release and slide your left foot toward you, over your right thigh. Place it on top of your right thigh with the sole facing up (6.14h). Tuck the heel in your right groin. Drop your left knee toward the floor.

Draw your thighs in toward each other and lengthen your spine from the base. Hook the points of your shoulder blades into your back, inhale, and lift and expand your chest. Spread your collarbones. Keep your spine perpendicular to the floor. Rest your hands on your thighs, palms facing up (6.14i).

To come out, support the left leg from beneath the shin and ankle and slide it away from you. Stretch the leg out in front of you. Support the leg that was underneath in a similar way, and return to Dandasana. Repeat the pose, bringing the left foot onto the right thigh first.

CAUTIONS. Great care should be taken not to invite injury in this or any other pose. Rather than force your knees, take all the time you need. It may take months or even years to systematically release the tightness in the hip joints. All it takes to injure your knees is one aggressive movement! Supta Padangusthasana III should not be practiced during menstruation because this is strenuous work and constricts the abdominal organs.

Padmasana is considered to be the best pose for meditation. Compared to the other sitting poses, it is easier to maintain a strong, stable, upward extension of the spine when the legs are locked in this pose. However, do not practice the pose for longer than a few minutes unless you are an experienced student.

ARDHA PADMASANA. If your legs do not slide easily into place, or if the first knee that you fold does not reach the floor, do not force them. In this case, you are not ready for Padmasana, so practice Ardha Padmasana. Tuck the second leg under the first leg, rather than over the first leg (6.14j).

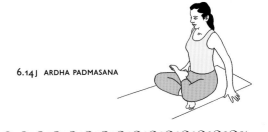

6.14J ARDHA PADMASANA

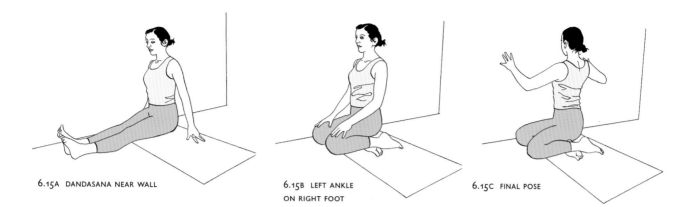

6.15A DANDASANA NEAR WALL

6.15B LEFT ANKLE ON RIGHT FOOT

6.15C FINAL POSE

6.15

Bharadvajasana
Bent-Knee Twist Pose with Wall

BENEFITS. When practicing Bharadvajasana, the spine undergoes a lateral rotation, which helps create both flexibility and strength. Tension is released in the shoulders and neck. Fat is reduced around the abdomen and waist, and the internal organs are toned and strengthened. This modification of the classic pose allows women to practice without straining the pelvic organs.

PRACTICE. With twists, you are playing with opposite forces. One part of the body is the stable foundation and does not move, and the other revolves away from the base.

Place a folded blanket on a mat, with the narrow side a few inches from the wall. Sit in Dandasana alongside a wall, with your right buttock on the folded blanket (6.15a). Sitting on a height facilitates a greater lift of the lower spine. With your thighs parallel to the wall, bend your legs and fold them to the left. Place your left ankle on top of the sole of the upturned right foot, so your left shin and right foot form a cross (6.15b). Turn

to the right, and place your hands, at shoulder height, on the wall (6.15c).

Press your left back ribs into your torso with an upward sweep. Keep that momentum going as you exhale and revolve your torso to the right. This movement of the back ribs, along with the gentle pressure of your fingertips on the wall, provides the support needed to lift and open the chest.

Check that your spine and torso are upright and perpendicular to the floor. Keep your left sit bone weighted toward the floor as you turn. Feel the whole length of the spine rotating. As you bring your breastbone to face the wall, lift and open your collarbones.

Do not push your lumbar forward. Do not hold for too long in the beginning. Do the pose quickly a few times first to get the spine moving.

To come out, release your bent knees and sit in Dandasana. Repeat the pose to the other side. When done, return to Dandasana.

CAUTIONS. Do not practice this pose if you have had recent abdominal or knee surgery, if you are menstruating, or if you are suffering from herniated or spinal disk injuries. Also avoid this pose if you have a migraine headache, high blood pressure, or diarrhea.

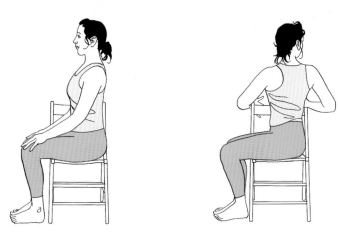

6.16A SIT SIDEWAYS ON THE CHAIR   6.16B FINAL POSE

6.16

Supported Bharadvajasana I
Chair-Twist Pose Sitting to the Side

BENEFITS. You can dispel exhaustion by practicing this pose. This gentle but effective twist is recommended for beginners and can also be used to relieve lower back pain. It makes the spine supple, exercises the abdominal muscles, and improves digestion.

PRACTICE. Sit sideways on the chair, with your left outer thigh parallel and close to the front edge of the chair and your feet 12 inches apart (6.16a). Hold the back of the chair with both hands. Sit up straight. Inhale and lift your side ribs and open your chest. With an exhalation, turn to the right, bringing the chest parallel to the back of the chair (6.16b).

Extend your inner right knee away from you to keep your knees level with each other. Use your hands to help you turn farther to the right; push with your left hand and pull with your right. Inhale, move your back ribs in, and lift; exhale and turn farther to the right. Lengthen through your left side ribs so that your collarbones and both sides of the chest are level with the floor.

To come out, turn your torso back to face your legs. Stand up. Sit facing the other way, so your right thigh lines up with the front of the chair. Repeat on this side.

CAUTIONS. It is particularly important for women to not push the lumbar spine into the abdominal region. Make sure that you have weight moving down over the left side of your sacrum, and take care that your belly does not roll forward. Do not practice this pose during menstruation or if you have a migraine headache, diarrhea, or high blood pressure.

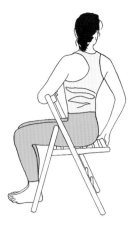

6.17A FINAL POSE

6.17

Supported Bharadvajasana II
Twist Sitting Backward through a Chair

BENEFITS. This pose provides a simple method of decompressing the lumbar vertebrae and releasing catches in the lower back. This variation is also valuable because the abdominal rotation can be controlled and restricted to some degree, in order to avoid over-squeezing the internal pelvic organs. This variation can be practiced during menstruation (provided the menstrual flow is not at its heaviest) to relieve low back pain, as it is not likely to cause the menstrual flow to increase.

PRACTICE. If practicing this pose after Viparita Dandasana II (10.2d), stay in your chair. Otherwise, climb through it and sit facing the chair back.

Place your left forearm on top of the chair rest. Hold the underneath of the chair seat with your right hand. Inhale and lift your chest. With an exhalation, turn to your right (6.17a). Roll your right shoulder back, release your shoulders away from your ears, and press your shoulder blades into your back. Feel the extension through both sides of your waist.

If you want to achieve a strong rotation in the lower back, press your right knee away from you, fix your hips firmly into the chair seat, and rotate strongly to the right. For a less extreme rotation, you can let the hips move with you a little as you twist, keeping the abdomen and waist relaxed (but lifted), and taking the twist into the upper torso. Make sure your spine is lifted up along its entire length as you turn.

To come out, turn your torso to face the back of the chair. Repeat on the other side.

CAUTIONS. Do not push forward into your belly or suck it back toward your lumbar spine as you turn. Do not practice this pose if you have a migraine headache, diarrhea, or high blood pressure.

Seated Forward Bends: Calming the Mind

W E TOUCH the quiet, reflective aspect of our consciousness when we practice forward bends. They calm the mind, soothe the nerves, and remove fatigue. In addition they stabilize blood pressure and pacify overworked adrenal glands. Forward bends are particularly restful around the time of menstruation, when feelings of frustration and irritability may be amplified. They reduce abdominal bloating and regularize blood sugar levels. When pelvic congestion inflames the nerve endings in the lower back, forward bends can relieve the pain.

Forward bends also break up abdominal hardness; when practiced correctly they relax the abdominal organs and help prevent the formation of fibroids. They also benefit those with oligomenorrhea (infrequent or delayed periods) and hypomenorrhea (scanty periods), by increasing the blood supply (and therefore oxygen and nutrients) to the ovaries and uterus, and by relieving mental stress. Additionally their practice reduces the possibility of irregular periods or an excessively heavy or prolonged menstrual flow. These poses are helpful when you are constipated or suffering from digestive problems.

A regular practice of the seated forward bends develops flexibility and fluidity of mind and body. However, before exploring them, first develop strength and stability through the practice of the standing poses, even if, like many women, you are already flexible. Practice this sequence for a few months before embarking on the seated forward bends: Uttanasana; Adho Mukha Svanasana; two or three standing poses, such as Utthita Trikonasana, Utthita Parsvakonasana, and Parsvottanasana; Halasana; Salamba Sarvangasana I.

Have patience: allow the process of releasing the hamstrings and gluteal muscles to take as long as it needs to. Eventually you will be able to bend forward from the hips, rather than from the waist, and your forward bends will become fluid and graceful.

General Cautions for Practicing Seated Forward Bends

When practicing the seated forward bends presented in this chapter, remember to follow these guidelines. Cautions are also included with each pose.

- During menstruation or if you are practicing to relieve premenstrual tension, support your head and remain in the pose for as long as you can, until the tension in the body dissolves. As you come to the end of menstruation and the flow gets lighter, reduce or dispense with the support.

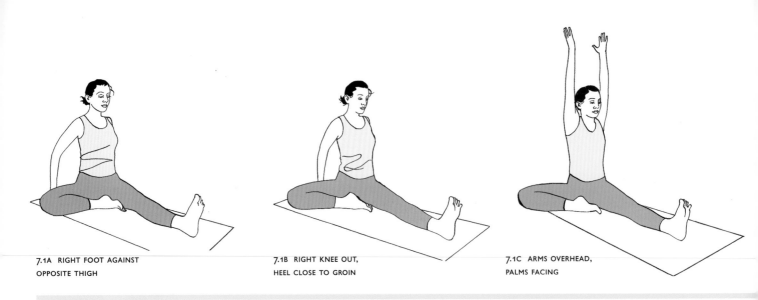

7.1A RIGHT FOOT AGAINST
OPPOSITE THIGH

7.1B RIGHT KNEE OUT,
HEEL CLOSE TO GROIN

7.1C ARMS OVERHEAD,
PALMS FACING

- Change sides frequently within the specified time if your hamstrings are so painful that your face, chest, or abdominal muscles get hard, or if your breathing becomes labored.

- Do not tense your abdomen. Lengthen and elongate your torso, without sucking in, gripping, or pushing into the abdomen.

- Do not practice seated forward bends if you are clinically or otherwise depressed, have a herniated disk, are feeling weepy from premenstrual tension, or have diarrhea.

- The forward bends are contraindicated during menstruation, when bleeding is excessive. However, Janu Sirsasana and Paschimottanasana can be practiced with the legs apart and a support under the head to great benefit.

- For some women, the hormonal shift that occurs just before menstruation (or ovulation) can result in a feeling of instability around the pelvis, especially if a weakness in the sacral ligaments already exists. Women with tight psoas muscles have told me that the sacrum and pelvis twist during the premenstrual phase. Whatever the cause, the hips can go out prior to menstruation. For these women, the deep forward extensions can exacerbate this condition. (Adho Mukha Upavista Konasana in particular

can aggravate an unstable pelvis.) Toward the end of the week following menstruation, things usually right themselves, and the standing poses will then help you feel more organized. However, if you feel that your sacroiliac joint shifts during menstruation, work carefully and mindfully in the forward bends. *Always* use support under your head at this time so you do not strain the lower back or pelvic joints.

7.1
Janu Sirsasana
Head-of-the-Knee Pose

BENEFITS. Janu Sirsasana tones the uterus and ovaries and helps them maintain hormonal balance. If your menstrual flow is prolonged or excessive, or if your periods are infrequent, painful, or scanty, regular practice of this pose will help bring the cycle back to normal. It can help reduce high blood pressure and soreness and bloating in the breasts or abdomen. This pose eases menstrual headaches and reduces food cravings as blood sugar levels stabilize. Janu Sirsasana also improves the circulation around the genitals and helps maintain vaginal health. The mind quiets when it is not projecting outward.

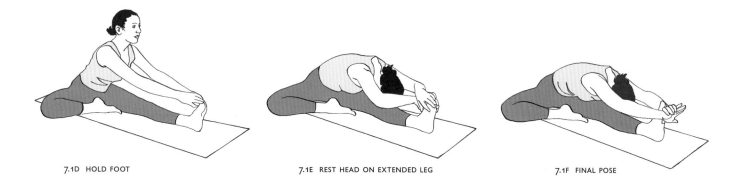

PRACTICE. Sit on your mat in Dandasana (6.1a) and bend your right knee out to the side. Keep the left leg straight and point the toes of the left foot toward the ceiling.

If you are a beginning student, place your right foot against the opposite thigh, and be careful not to push your hips out of alignment (7.1a). If you are a continuing student, fold your right knee as far out to the side as possible, and draw your right heel close in to your right groin (7.1b). Turn your right foot outward, from the pinky to the big toe, so the sole of the foot faces the ceiling,

Place your hands behind you and press your fingertips into the floor. Draw your sacrum in and up, and lift your side ribs. Revolve your torso to the left, lining up the center of your breastbone with the inner edge of your left leg.

Inhale and raise your arms over your head with the palms facing each other (7.1c). Lift up evenly through both sides of your torso and press your shoulder blades into your back. Bending forward from the hips and leading with your breastbone, exhale and catch hold of your left foot with both hands.

Bring your shoulder blades into contact with your upper back. Use them to help you curve your thoracic spine in, so the lumbar spine lengthens. Raise your head and lift and open your chest (7.1d).

Much of the power of this asymmetrical pose is generated by striving for symmetry. Keep your bent leg firmly in contact with the floor, and roll your navel over the left thigh. Extend the inner walls of the abdomen evenly on both sides.

Now bring the head down: With an exhalation, extend forward and rest your head on your left (extended) leg (7.1e). Keep your neck relaxed and your eyes and head quiet throughout. Avoid constricting the chest or tensing the abdomen. Bend your elbows out. Release your shoulders away from your neck and lengthen the armpits. If you can easily hold your foot, turn your hands out and clasp your right wrist with your left hand (7.1f).

If you experience pain in your hamstrings, then change sides frequently, but know that ultimately the longer you stay in the pose, the more cooling and calming the effect. To come out, inhale and raise your head and curve your spine up. Release your hands and sit up. Return to Dandasana, and repeat on the other side.

CAUTIONS. If you have had a back injury or are experiencing back pain, do not take the head down. When menstruating, pass briefly through the first stage of the pose, where the head is up. The focus at this time is to relax into the pose with the brain quiet and the head supported.

第14贴　正面 凯源-4色-WomandYoga-内页拼版.job

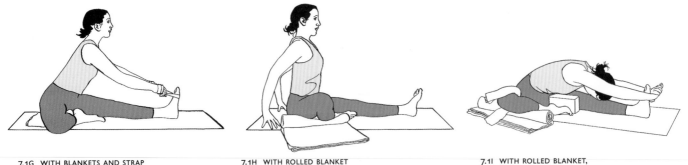

7.1G WITH BLANKETS AND STRAP   7.1H WITH ROLLED BLANKET   7.1I WITH ROLLED BLANKET, WASHCLOTH, AND BLOCK

JANU SIRSASANA WITH BLANKETS AND STRAP. If you are unable to hold your foot, place one or more folded blankets under your hips, slip a belt around your outstretched foot, and hold it with both hands (7.1g).

JANU SIRSANANA WITH ROLLED BLANKET. If you feel strain in your bent knee or it does not touch the floor, then support it with a rolled blanket (7.1h).

JANU SIRSASANA WITH ROLLED BLANKET, WASH-CLOTH, AND BLOCK. Tight hips can cause knee problems. To open the hip joint and, at the same time, protect the knee, place a rolled blanket under it and a folded washcloth behind it. Then position a block between your bent-knee foot and the inside of your extended leg. Press your foot against the block and extend through the inner knee of your bent leg (7.1i).

JANU SIRSANSANA WITH CHAIR. If your forehead does not rest easily on your leg or a bolster, or if you feel pain in the back of your legs, rest your head on a chair (7.1j). Do not be discouraged! Persistent practice eventually results in the hamstrings lengthening and the forward bend deepening. If you have uterine fibroids or a migraine headache or are experiencing a heavy flow, you

will find it more comfortable and more beneficial to work this way.

JANU SIRSASANA WITH HORIZONTAL BOLSTER. During your period or if you are experiencing premenstrual tension, practice this pose passively. Do not take the bent leg back so far, even if you are experienced in the pose. And at this time, always use support under your head, and place one or more blankets under your hips. Place a bolster (or folded blanket) horizontally across your shin (7.1k). Working this way also releases abdominal tension, making it less likely for fibroids to form.

JANU SIRSASANA WITH VERTICAL BOLSTER AND BLANKETS. If you experience lower back pain or abdominal cramping, place a bolster (or folded blanket) lengthwise along your leg and rest your belly over the support. Place one or more folded blankets across the bolster for your head to rest on (7.1l). Experiment to see which method you prefer (a horizontal bolster, as in 7.1k, or a vertical bolster). There should be no muscular exertion during menstruation.

JANU SIRSASANA WITH LEGS APART. During the heaviest phase of your period, or if you have a headache or high blood pressure or suffer from

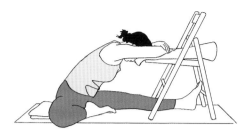

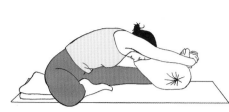

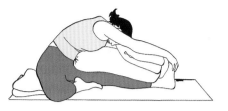

obesity, it will be more soothing and more comfortable to practice this asana with the legs apart. Swing your left (extended) leg out 12 inches to the left. Extend your rib cage forward and support your head on a bolster (or chair) (7.1m).

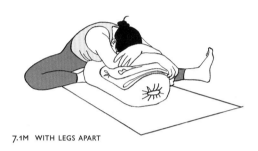

7.1M WITH LEGS APART

7.2

Triang Mukhaikapada Paschimottanasana
Half-Hero in Seated Forward Bend Pose

BENEFITS. Each of the forward bends in this chapter stimulates the circulation in the pelvis in its own unique way. Triang Mukhaikapada Paschimottanasana tones the liver, and a well-functioning liver is essential for efficient detoxification. The pose also improves flexibility in the knee and ankle joints, and it calms the mind.

PRACTICE. The stability of this pose comes from careful positioning at the base. To begin, sit on your mat in Dandasana (6.1a). Fold your right leg back and place a folded blanket under your left sitting bone (7.2a). Keep your right shin and foot close into your right thigh, and check that your thighs are parallel to each other. Make space behind your bent knee; with your hands, roll your right calf muscle out. Extend through your inner left foot and spread your toes.

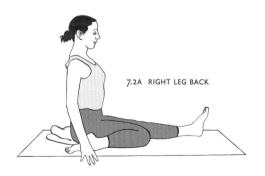

7.2A RIGHT LEG BACK

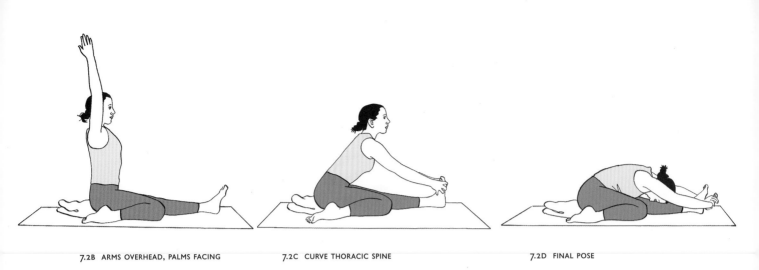

7.2B ARMS OVERHEAD, PALMS FACING   7.2C CURVE THORACIC SPINE   7.2D FINAL POSE

The grounding of the bent-leg sitting bone comes with practice. Roll your left thigh in. With your hand, draw your left buttock flesh out and sit on the center of your left sitting bone. Press your fingertips into the floor at either side of your hips. Press your right buttock down and bring your weight to the center of your pelvis. Inhale and lift your spine from the base of the pelvis. Open your chest and spread your collarbones from the center out.

Inhale and raise your arms overhead with your palms facing in (7.2b). Lift evenly through both sides of your torso and press your shoulder blades into your back. Exhale and extend your torso forward, and take hold of your left foot with both hands.

Broaden through the ball of the left foot and press it out into your hands. Press your left thigh down. Raise the sides of the chest. Curve your thoracic spine in and up (7.2c). Extend from the pubis to the throat. Roll your shoulders back and raise your head.

Bending your elbows out to the sides, extend your torso along your left thigh, without creating any tension in the abdomen. Place your head on your shin (7.2d).

Remain balanced on the center of your sitting bones. Spread your left toes and broaden through the ball of your left foot. Shift the weight of the torso to the right to avoid tipping to the left. Allow your back ribs to soften and release. If you can reach farther with your hands, turn your palms away from you and clasp your left wrist with your right hand.

To come out, inhale and raise your head, curving your spine up. Release your hands and sit up. Return your legs to Dandasana. Repeat on the other side.

CAUTIONS. If you have a knee injury, seek the advice of an experienced yoga teacher before attempting this pose. During menstruation, pass briefly through the first stage of the pose, where the head is up. Practice the pose quietly and with support; focus on the soft release of the torso as it extends forward over the bolster (or folded blanket) and on the head resting quietly Avoid this pose during menstruation if you are bleeding profusely, are bleeding between periods, or if you have ovarian cysts, endometriosis, fibroids, or migraine headache. If you have a lower back injury, practice only with the head up and the spine concave (7.2c).

TRIANG MUKHAIKAPADA PASCHIMOTTANASANA WITH STRAP. If you are unable to take hold of your

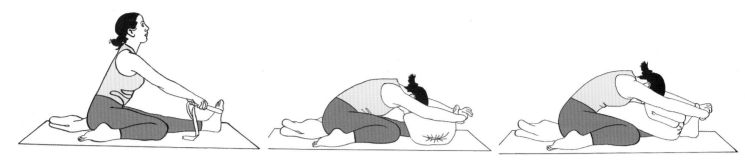

7.2E WITH STRAP   7.2F WITH HORIZONTAL BOLSTER   7.2G WITH VERTICAL BOLSTER

foot in the first stage of the pose, where the head is up, place a strap around your foot and hold both ends, one in each hand (7.2e).

TRIANG MUKHAIKAPADA PASCHIMOTTANASANA WITH HORIZONTAL BOLSTER. If you are menstruating, if your head does not reach your leg, or if you feel pain in the extended leg, rest your head on a bolster (or chair) and place one or more blankets under your hips (7.2f).

TRIANG MUKHAIKAPADA PASCHIMOTTANASANA WITH VERTICAL BOLSTER. If you experience low back pain or abdominal cramps during your period, practice with a bolster (or folded blanket) placed vertically, along your extended leg and a folded blanket under your forehead (7.2g)

7·3
Ardha Padma Paschimottanasana
Half-Lotus in Seated Forward Bend Pose

BENEFITS. Ardha Padma Paschimottanasana improves the circulation in the pelvic cavity and tones the abdominal organs. It increases mobility in the hips, knees, and ankles. It calms the mind and relaxes the senses.

PRACTICE. Sit on your mat in Dandasana (6.1a). Bend your right knee and hold your shin from underneath with your left hand (7.3a). Place your right foot onto the top of your left thigh.

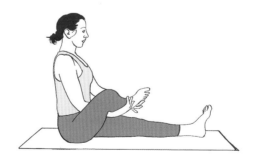

7.3A HOLD SHIN

第15贴　正面 凯源-4色-WomandYoga-内页拼版.job

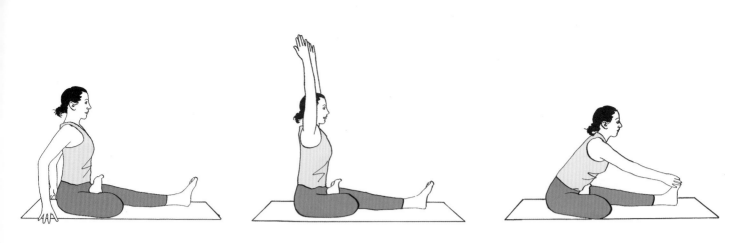

7.3B FINGERTIPS BESIDE HIPS   7.3C ARMS OVERHEAD, PALMS FACING   7.3D HOLD FOOT

If your foot has a tendency to slide off the receiving thigh or presses uncomfortably into it, come out of the pose and begin again. This time work more consciously to release the right hip. Swing your right thigh out to the right and externally rotate your right thigh deep within its socket before drawing the heel in toward the navel again. Then bring your foot high onto your left thigh. With patient and persistent practice, the hips become more flexible, and this procedure gets easier.

Sit on the front of your sitting bones. Extend the left leg, and center it on the midline of the left calf and thigh, so your kneecap faces straight up. Press your fingertips into the floor beside your hips, inhale, and raise your spine and open your chest (7.3b). Inhale again and raise your arms overhead, with your palms facing each other (7.3c). Lift evenly through both sides of your torso and press your shoulder blades into your back. Fully stretch your arms. Exhale, fold forward from the pelvis, and reach out to hold your left foot with both hands (7.3d).

Press the inner edge of your left foot out into your hands and press your left thigh down. Curve your thoracic spine forward and up, expand your chest, and raise your head (7.3e). Roll your shoulders back. Spread your collarbones out from the center. Remember not to suck or grip the abdomen in toward the spine.

Then proceed to the next stage of the pose: maintaining the openness of your chest, exhale, and fold forward over your left (extended) leg. Rest your head on your shin.

Slide your abdomen farther along your left leg and relax the belly as you do this. Release your spine downward and extend your arms out from your shoulders. If you can reach farther with your hands, turn your hands out and catch hold of your wrist (7.3f).

To come out, raise your head and curve your spine up. Release your grasp on the left foot, inhale, and sit up. Undo the folded leg. Return to Dandasana, and repeat the pose on the other side.

CAUTIONS. You must come into this pose very carefully. The mobility of the bent leg comes from the flexibility of the hip joint. *Never* force your knees or ask them to do the work of the hips. When you are menstruating, pass briefly through the first stage of the pose, where the head is up and the spine concave, and then practice the second stage in Ardha Padma Paschimottanasana with Horizontal Bolster or Chair (7.3i and 7.3j). Do not practice this pose, even supported, if you have heavy periods, are bleeding between periods, or have ovarian cysts, endometriosis, or fibroid tumors. Do not practice this pose if you have had recent knee surgery or have a herniated disk.

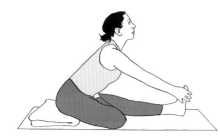

7.3E LOOK UP

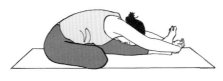

7.3F FINAL POSE

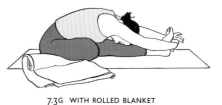

7.3G WITH ROLLED BLANKET

Ardha Padma Paschimottanasana with Rolled Blanket. If your bent knee does not touch the floor, place a firmly rolled blanket under the bent knee (7.3g)

Ardha Padma Paschimottanasana with Strap. If you are unable to take hold of your foot, place a strap around your foot and hold both ends, one in each hand, and place one or more blankets under the hips (7.3h)

Ardha Padma Paschimottanasana with Horizontal Bolster or Chair. If restricted mobility around the hips and pelvis prevents your head from reaching your shin, rest your head on a bolster (7.3i) or on a chair (7.3j). You can place one or more folded blankets under your hips to release the abdomen even more and to take you further into the forward bend.

Ardha Padma Paschimottanasana with Vertical Bolster. If you experience low back pain or abdominal cramps, try working with a bolster (or folded blanket) placed along the extended leg and a folded blanket under your forehead (7.3k).

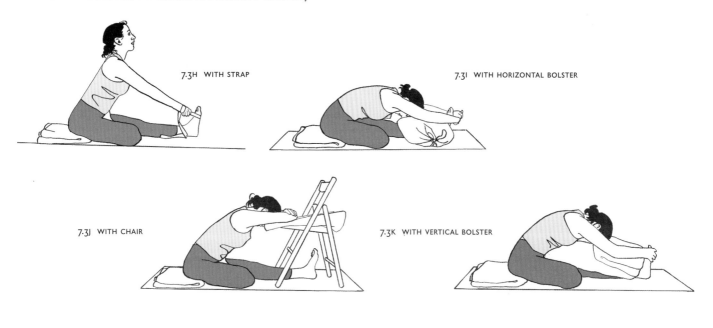

7.3H WITH STRAP

7.3I WITH HORIZONTAL BOLSTER

7.3J WITH CHAIR

7.3K WITH VERTICAL BOLSTER

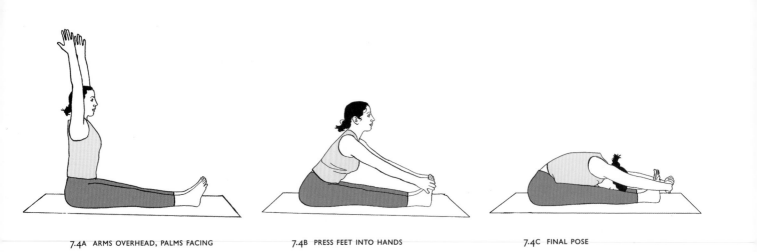

7.4A ARMS OVERHEAD, PALMS FACING   7.4B PRESS FEET INTO HANDS   7.4C FINAL POSE

7·4

Paschimottanasana
Seated Forward Bend Pose

BENEFITS. Paschimottanasana lengthens the spine and stretches the hamstrings. The pelvic organs are supplied with an abundant flow of blood and *prana,* or life force, and problems caused by sluggish digestion, including constipation, are eliminated. This pose also stimulates the entire reproductive system. Most important, it induces a peaceful state of mind.

PRACTICE. Sit in Dandasana (6.1a). Roll the tops of your thighs in and use your hands to draw the flesh of the buttocks out. Fully stretch your legs. Press your fingertips down by your sides and, against that resistance, inhale and lengthen your spine.

Raise your arms above your head, palms facing inward, to create a dynamic extension through the waist, breasts, and shoulders (7.4a). Leading with your breastbone, reach forward and hold the sides of your feet. Spread your toes, broaden the balls of the feet and press your feet into your hands (7.4b).

Roll your shoulders back and down and straighten your arms. Curve your thoracic spine in and up and lift your side ribs. Spread your collarbones out from the center. Your chest should feel full and open. As in all sitting forward bends, relax your neck and keep your head passive and your eyes quiet. Raise your head and look up. Then, maintaining the lift of the chest, exhale and fold forward from the hips. Rest your abdomen, chest, and head on your legs (7.4c).

To intensify the fold from the hips, draw your thigh muscles back toward your groins and move your sitting bones back. Using your side ribs, not your spine, exhale and extend your torso farther forward and up. Raise your elbows to create length in the armpits and side ribs and open the shoulder joints. If you can easily hold your feet, turn your hands out and clasp your left wrist with your right hand. To come out, release your hands, inhale, and return to Dandasana.

CAUTIONS. If you are menstruating, pass briefly through the head-up stage of the pose. Support your head so that the abdomen and chest remain free and extended, and the brain quiet. Do not practice with the head down if you have herniated or bulging disks; practice as in figure 7.4b.

PASCHIMOTTANASANA WITH STRAP. If your back is rounded when you bend forward and reach your

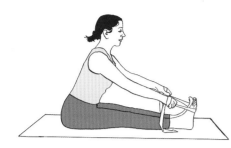

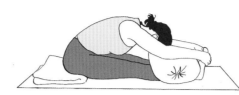

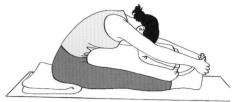

7.4D WITH STRAP

7.4E WITH HORIZONTAL BOLSTER

7.4F WITH VERTICAL BOLSTER

feet, or if you cannot hold your feet, place a strap around your feet and curve your spine in (7.4d).

PASCHIMOTTANASANA WITH HORIZONTAL BOLSTER. If you are menstruating or if you head does not rest easily on the shins, support your head on a horizontal bolster (or a folded blanket) and place one or more blankets under your hips (7.4e). The weight of the support helps the legs to release toward the floor, which further encourages the uterine muscles to relax.

PASCHIMOTTANASANA WITH VERTICAL BOLSTER. If you experience lower back pain or abdominal cramps, try working with a bolster (or folded blanket) placed along the extended leg and a folded blanket under your forehead(7.4f).

PASCHIMOTTTANASANA WITH LEGS APART AND BOLSTER OR CHAIR. Those with fibroids, ovarian cysts, blocked fallopian tubes, problems with the menstrual flow, or who are overweight will benefit by sitting on one (or more) folded blankets, and practicing with the legs hip-width apart and the head resting on a bolster (7.4g) or chair seat (7.4h).

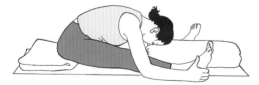

7.4G WITH LEGS APART AND BOLSTER

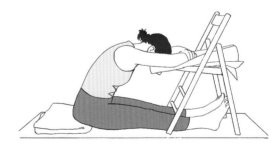

7.4H WITH LEGS APART AND CHAIR

Reclining Poses: Restoring Lost Energy

WE SEEM TO BE sacrificing more and more of our time and energy to our high-speed culture and, as a consequence, exhaustion and depression have become familiar aspects of life. Traditionally women are the nurturers and caregivers in society. But all too often we forget to take care of ourselves.

Deciding that you are important and making room in your frantic schedule for some downtime are important steps toward self-care. By far the most effective method of replenishing energy is to practice restorative yoga. It can leave you feeling refreshed and ready for life again. And a restorative yoga sequence doesn't have to be very long.

At first glance these poses may not look dramatic or challenging. But each pose is deeply therapeutic and helps to release tension and restore energy. These poses are powerfully nurturing, in part because they can be held for longer than most other postures because the body is supported. They cool an agitated brain, reduce elevated blood pressure, rest the nervous system, and enable the immune and endocrine systems to function more efficiently.

Reclining poses can be practiced actively or passively, depending on the desired outcome.

During menstruation, when the body and mind need to be quiet and still, practice them in a restful way with a minimum of effort. The reclining poses are particularly helpful for dealing with menstrual dysfunction. For example, by regularly letting go of abdominal and nervous tension in Supta Baddha Konasana II, an excessively heavy menstrual flow can be greatly reduced. Cramps can also be relieved by practicing these poses. Surrender yourself fully to each pose and discover for yourself what each one has to teach you.

General Cautions for Practicing the Reclining Poses

When practicing the reclining poses presented in this chapter, remember to follow these guidelines. Cautions are also included with each pose.

■ Do not practice the reclining poses if you have had recent abdominal surgery.

■ If you wear contact lenses or glasses, remove them at the start of any practice session that includes reclining poses.

■ If you have low blood pressure, keep yourself warm by covering up.

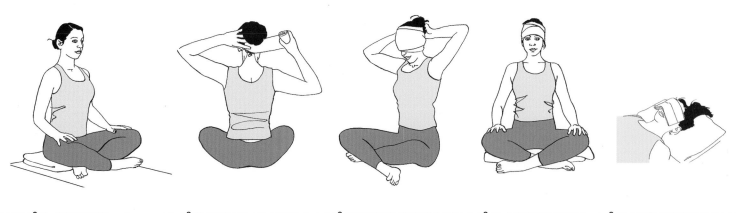

8.1

Head Wrapping

BENEFITS. Your mind is less likely to obsess over problems when you wrap the head, ears, and eyes with a bandage. The wrap ensures that the eyes and ears are passive, the facial muscles relax, mental tension is relieved, and the nerves are soothed. It is helpful to work with the head wrapped if you have insomnia and when practicing pranayama.

WRAPPING THE HEAD AND EYES. Sit in Swastikasana (8.1a). Hold the bandage roll in your right hand, with the roll facing away from you and the tail in your left hand. Hold the tail against the back of your head and, slowly unraveling the roll, wrap it around your head in a counterclockwise direction (8.1b). Wrap it over your right ear.

Draw the head wrap across your forehead, from right to left, above your eyes. Take it around your left ear, and pass it behind your skull again. On the second and subsequent passes, completely cover your ears and eyes. When you get to the end, tuck the tail securely into the folds of the head wrap (8.1c).

WRAPPING THE FOREHEAD. Beginners can familiarize themselves with this practice by wrapping only the forehead. This is also recommended for those with migraine headaches; the pressure of the bandage helps the blood vessels in the scalp deflate and cool down.

Wrap the head in a similar manner, but do not cover the eyes. Do cover the eyebrows (8.1d). Alternatively, when you have settled into a reclining pose, place a bandage folded (to about 7 inches in length) or a small folded towel lightly over your eyes (8.1e).

HOW TO UNWRAP. When finished, turn to your side. If you are practicing with the bandage folded over your eyes, simply let if fall off. Sit up in Swastikasana. If you have the bandage wrapped around your head, then slowly unwind the bandage from your head and drop it into your lap. Now calmly and deliberately reroll it. This action brings you back into the world and allows the senses to slowly reemerge from within in a way that does not disturb the nerves.

CAUTIONS. Do not compress the head or eyes by wrapping the bandage too tightly. Do not tuck the bandage in at the back of the head, as this will interfere with the placement of the skull.

If you wrap the bandage firmly but so it is com-

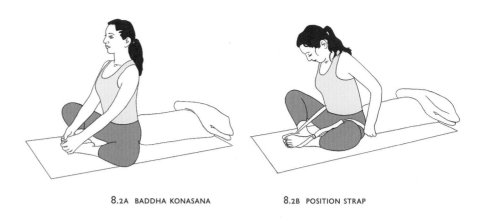

8.2A BADDHA KONASANA   8.2B POSITION STRAP

fortable for your eyes and forehead, it should stay in place until you decide to undo it. While you are setting up at the start of your practice or between poses, fold the bandage up off your eyes so you can see. Fold it down again as you settle into each new pose.

8.2
Supta Baddha Konasana I
Reclining Bound-Angle Pose I

BENEFITS. Many of Western women's reproductive and digestive problems stem from abdominal tension. The primary physical benefits of this pose are a soft, relaxed belly and healthy abdominal organs. Practice it during your period, especially if you suffer from menstrual cramps or when your energy levels are low. The abdominal fatigue and pelvic soreness that sometimes accompany menstruation are also alleviated. In addition, this pose has a "drying" effect on the internal organs and helps to reduce a heavy menstrual flow and diarrhea.

Some women have cystitis (burning sensations when urinating and frequency of urination) around the time of menstruation. This pose relaxes the bladder and can help to relieve these symptoms. Finally, Supta Baddha Konasana I improves circulation in the chest, releases tension in the diaphragm, and softens the breath. Practice this pose before pranayama (see chapters 11 and 14) to calm the mind and expand and relax the lungs.

PRACTICE. Place a bolster along the center of your mat, and one or more blankets, sufficient to support your head, at the top end of the bolster. Sit in Baddha Konasana, with the blankets and bolster behind you (8.2a). To prevent your feet from sliding way, secure them with a strap: start with the strap open and pass it under your feet, over your ankles and thighs, and around your lower back. Fasten the buckle. Make sure the strap rests at your tailbone. Tighten the strap, drawing your heels close to your pelvis (8.2b). Lower your torso back onto the bolster.

When the head is thrown back or the chin is lifted, the throat becomes tense and the brain agitated. To position your head correctly, first make sure that the blanket completely supports your head and neck, not your shoulders. Then interlace your fingers behind your neck and slide your hands toward the crown of your head, so the back of the neck lengthens. Your head should be centered and supported so it does not tip to the side.

To elongate the abdominal muscles and mas-

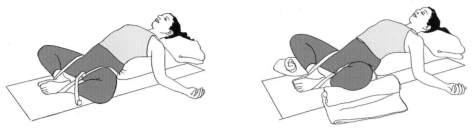

8.2C FINAL POSE   8.2D WITH ROLLED BLANKETS

sage the pelvic organs, start by folding your arms above your head. After a minute or two, rest your arms on the floor and at your sides (8.2c). Roll your shoulders back away from your ears, and lift and open your chest.

To be effective, the restorative poses require an attitude of receptivity and surrender. Willpower plays no part in their practice. Allow your lower back to settle into the support. Soften your eyes, release your lower jaw, and relax your tongue so it rests lightly on your lower palate. Allow a sense of length to come to your neck, and relax your throat. Let the ribs and collarbones open outward. Feel the openness of the chest, and let the heart center be receptive. Notice how your whole body has softened. Relax the groins and open to the healing energy filling the womb, the fallopian tubes, and the ovaries. Allow your breath to flow easily and your mind to rest. Be completely absorbed into the posture.

To come out, raise your knees with your hands. Slip your feet out of the strap. Use your hands to push up to a seated position. That way, strain on the abdomen and lumbar spine is minimized.

CAUTIONS. Do not practice this pose or its variations if you have a lower back injury or persistent lower back pain.

SUPTA BADDHA KONASANA I WITH ROLLED BLANKETS. If the stretch of the inner groins and thighs prevents you from relaxing, support them with the firmly rolled blankets (8.2d). Rolled blankets placed under the knees also helps reduce low back strain in this pose. Women who suffer from an excessively heavy menstrual flow due to fibroids often experience tightness across the uterus during menstruation, and the rolled blankets under the knees reduces the pull.

SUPTA BADDHA KONASANA I WITH FOLDED BLANKET. If you experience lower back pain, slide a little farther away from the bolster. If this does not alleviate the pain, decrease the height of your support. Similarly if you have fibroids, you may want to reduce the height of the support from a bolster to one (or two) folded blankets, to minimize abdominal pressure (8.2e).

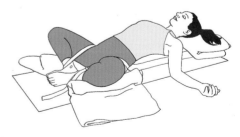

8.2E WITH FOLDED BLANKET

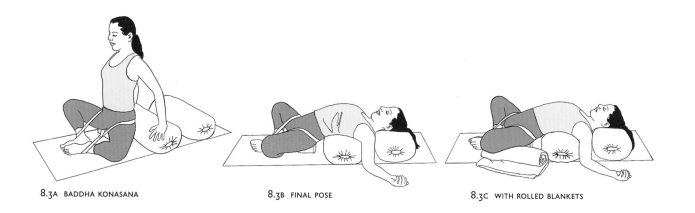

8.3A BADDHA KONASANA   8.3B FINAL POSE   8.3C WITH ROLLED BLANKETS

8.3

Supta Baddha Konasana II
Reclining Bound-Angle Pose II

BENEFITS. All the versions of Supta Baddha Konasana promote health for the uterine and urinary systems. In both my practice and teaching experience, this version never fails to soothe menstrual pain. The elevation of the pelvis pacifies and relaxes the pelvic area. This variation is helpful in correcting a displaced uterus. It is an effective remedy for exhaustion, low blood pressure, abdominal fatigue, and menstrual cramps. In addition it can reduce a heavy menstrual flow and the symptoms of diarrhea (during menstruation or at any other time) and can soothe swollen or tender breasts.

PRACTICE. Position two bolsters across the end of your mat, with the long sides parallel and approximately two inches apart.

Sit on a block in Baddha Konasana, facing away from the bolsters, and secure your feet with a strap (8.3a). Coil your back ribs in and curve back over the first bolster. Allow your shoulders to roll down into the space between the two bolsters. Rest your head and neck on the second bol-

ster. Rotate your upper arms outward in their sockets and rest your arms out to the sides, with your palms facing the ceiling (8.3b).

Be attentive to the sensations in the pelvis as they present themselves. First and foremost, quiet your mind and try not to bring your worries and preoccupations into this practice. Relax the face muscles. Then slide your tailbone toward your heels. Relax the sacrum, and feel it releasing and widening. Explore the length that is created in the muscles of the lower back. Soften the lower abdomen, soften the buttocks, relax the genitals (both inside and outside), and relax the inner thighs. Feel the spaciousness of the womb. Allow fear, pain, and discomfort to melt away from the soft tissues within your pelvis. Breathe evenly and naturally.

To come out, raise your legs a little and slip off the strap. Bend your knees and rest your feet on the floor. Raise your pelvis, and remove the block. Turn to your side and sit up.

CAUTIONS. Do not practice this pose or its variations if you have a lower back injury or persistent lower back pain.

SUPTA BADDHA KONASANA II WITH ROLLED BLANKETS. If your inner thighs start to feel tight, support them with rolled blankets (8.3c).

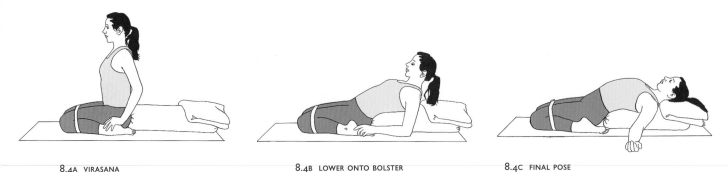

8.4A VIRASANA   8.4B LOWER ONTO BOLSTER   8.4C FINAL POSE

8.4

Supta Virasana
Reclining Hero's Pose

BENEFITS. By altering the flow of blood and releasing tension in the pelvic and abdominal regions, Supta Virasana brings healing energy to the digestive and urinary systems. It can help relieve acidity, stomachache, and cystitis. Menstrual problems stemming from disorders of the ovaries and inflammation of the reproductive organs are eased. It also soothes menstrual cramps and can help to correct a displaced uterus.

You can include this pose in your practice if you are feeling tired or to relax the nerves. Regular practice lengthens the psoas, the deep inner muscles that attach the spine to the upper thighbones. This allows the diaphragm and the abdominal muscles to relax, which in turn releases the inner organs towards the spine. As Geeta S. Iyengar points out in *Yoga: A Gem for Women*, this pose removes fatigue in the legs and improves the flexibility of the knees and ankles.

PRACTICE. At first, this pose may feel awkward. Don't be in a hurry to master it. Have patience: it may take time for the muscles to release and

the joints to become mobile enough for the pose to feel comfortable. Place a bolster along the center of your mat and one or more blankets, sufficient to support your head at the top end of your bolster.

Sit on your mat in Virasana, with the inner edges of your feet touching your hips (8.4a). Press the center of our feet and ankles against the floor. Draw your knees close to each other. If your thighs are not parallel to each other, wrap a strap around your shins and thighbones. If you are a beginning student, be aware that your body is not toned, and that strapping the knees too tightly can result in lower back strain.

Support your weight with your hands and, one at a time, lean back onto your elbows (8.4b). Coil your back ribs in and lift and open your chest. Lower yourself back onto the bolster.

Position your head carefully so it rests at the center and does not tip to one side: draw the blanket into position under your head and neck. Interlace your hands behind your head and gently lengthen your neck; place the head so the forehead slopes slightly down toward the chest and your throat relaxes.

Rest your arms at your sides, palms facing up, to expand the chest and deepen the breath. Turn your upper arms out at their sockets, and roll your shoulders away from your ears. Slide your shoul-

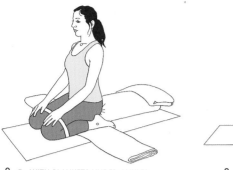

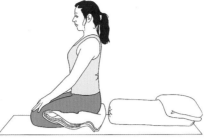

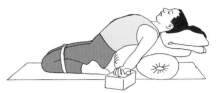

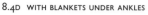

8.4D WITH BLANKETS UNDER ANKLES

8.4E WITH BLANKETS
BETWEEN THIGHS AND CALVES

8.4F WITH TWO BOLSTERS
AND BLOCKS

der blades toward your lower back, and lift your chest toward your head (8.4c).

Settle the buttock bones. Descend the tops of the thighbones toward the floor. To prevent your lumbar spine from overarching or compressing and becoming uncomfortable, raise your pelvis up and tuck your tailbone toward your heels.

Observe the inner walls of the pelvis, and allow the abdomen to release and soften. Allow the spine to elongate, the abdominal muscles to lengthen, and the chest to expand. Feel your torso completely supported as you release into the pose.

To come out, place your hands on the soles of your feet, roll your trapezius muscles (the muscles over your shoulder blades) toward your waist, and allow your upper back to support you as you inhale and sit up. Remove the strap. Slide your feet out to one side and stretch your legs out in front of you.

If your knees feel stiff, interlock your fingers and, one at a time, support the back of your thigh and stretch your leg out. Turn over onto one side and push up to standing. Alternatively drop your hands forward and stretch back into Adho Mukha Svanasana (5.5d). Step your feet forward and in between your hands, and come into Uttanasana (5.4c). Place your hands on your waist, inhale, and stand up.

CAUTIONS. If, despite the adjustments, your knees hurt, come out of the pose and wait for a few days before trying the pose again. When you resume practice of this pose, do not hold it for longer than 1 minute.

You should feel comfortable in Virasana (6.8c) and should be able to practice it without sitting on a block before you attempt Supta Virasana. Do not practice Supta Virasana during menstruation if you are bleeding excessively.

SUPTA VIRASANA WITH BLANKETS. If you experience ankle pain, place a folded blanket under them (8.4d). If you experience knee pain in the pose, place a folded blanket between the calves and the backs of the thighs (8.4e).

SUPTA VIRASANA WITH TWO BOLSTERS AND BLOCKS. If you find it difficult to lower your torso onto the support, add height by placing a second bolster, horizontally, underneath the first and your hands on blocks (8.4f).

SUPTA VIRASANA WITH DECREASED TORSO SUPPORT. For women with uterine fibroids, the abdominal stretch in this pose can be uncomfortable and may create stress around the uterus. Also some women report that during menstruation, on coming out of this pose, the menstrual flow

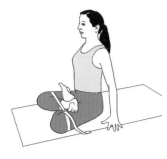

8.5A PADMASANA WITH STRAP

8.5B ARDHA PADMASANA
WITH STRAP (ALTERNATIVE)

8.5C LIE BACK, ARMS OVERHEAD

increases. As a result of practicing the pose, it may be that the uterus is able to expel clots from the uterine wall. If this happens, decrease the support under the torso, so you experience less of an arch in the lumbar spine. For example, place a folded blanket under your torso (8.4g).

SUPTA VIRASANA WITH ARMS ABOVE HEAD. Stretching the arms over the head helps relieve bloating and tenderness in the breasts and abdomen. Fold your arms above your head and rest them on your folded blanket (8.4h).

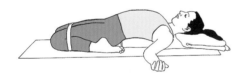

8.4G WITH DECREASED TORSO SUPPORT

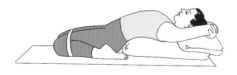

8.4H WITH ARMS ABOVE HEAD

8.5
Matsyasana
Fish Pose

BENEFITS. A reclining version of Padmasana, Matsyasana is an effective way of bringing life and flexibility into the hip joints and pelvis. It tones the abdominal muscles and pelvic organs. It counteracts the buildup of the tension that may contribute to the development of fibroid tumors and uterine and ovarian cysts. It also helps relieve hemorrhoids.

PRACTICE. Prepare your hips and knees by practicing Supta Padangusthasana III (6.14a through 6.14d). To practice Matsyasana, sit on your mat in Padmasana (8.5a) or Ardha Padmasana (8.5b). Hold Padmasana or Ardha Padmasana for only 10 seconds, twice on each side, before coming into Matsyasana (or Ardha Mastsyasana).

Secure a strap around your lower thighs (do not pull the strap too tight if you have problem knees). Lean back onto your elbows, coil your back ribs in, and lie back on your mat. Extend your arms over your head and rest them on the floor (8.5c).

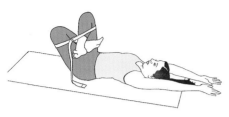

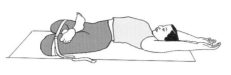

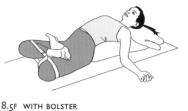

8.5D RAISE KNEES

8.5E FINAL POSE

8.5F WITH BOLSTER

Raise your knees until your thighs are perpendicular to the floor (8.5d). Activate your buttock muscles by squeezing your tailbone in. With an exhalation, extend your knees away and slowly bring your legs down to the floor (8.5e). Take care that you don't force this movement; allow it to be a process of release. The more you let go around the hip sockets and inner groins, the farther down toward the floor your legs will go. If, after this work, your knees do not touch to the floor, practice Matsyasana with Bolster instead (8.5f).

To come out, hold the sides of the mat, press your elbows into the floor, inhale, and sit up. Remove the strap. Release each leg out, one at a time, in the order that you took the pose. Sit in Dandasana (6.1a). Interlace your fingers behind your thighs, and extend each leg out through your heels to bring space back into the knee joint. Do this each time you change sides, as well as after you have finished in the pose. You can also come into Padmasana and exit Padmasana from the prone position.

CAUTIONS. *Always* prepare your knees and hips before coming into Padmasana or Ardha Padmasana. Postpone your practice of these poses if you have sore or swollen knees or have a knee injury.

MATSYASANA WITH BOLSTER. The supported version of this pose relieves stomachaches, acidity, and indigestion. It stretches the abdomen and waist and boosts the circulation of blood in the pelvic area. If you can practice Padmasana (8.5a) or Ardha Padmasana (8.5b) with ease, then practice Matsyasana with Bolster during menstruation to calm the mind, soothe the nerves, and relax the abdomen. Support your torso with a bolster and your head with a folded blanket. Rest your arms out to the sides (8.5f). If you experience abdominal tension, then place a rolled blanket under your knees (8.5g).

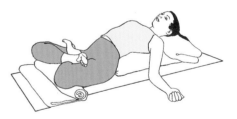

8.5G WITH BLANKET ROLL

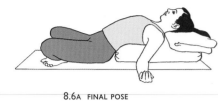

8.6A FINAL POSE

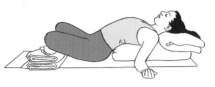

8.6B WITH BLANKETS

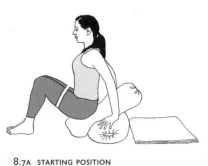

8.7A STARTING POSITION

8.6

Supta Swastikasana
Reclining Simple Cross-Leg Pose

BENEFITS. It is easier to relax by practicing several reclining poses rather than one long Savasana (8.14d) when your practice has not been vigorous, such as during menstruation. The reclining poses, particularly those where the legs are folded, have an immediately calming effect on the body and the nerves. Savasana, which involves much disciplined focus of attention, comes easier after a workout.

Practiced over a bolster, Supta Swastikasana opens the chest and the emotional center. It relieves stiffness in the back and creates movement and freedom through the pelvic joints. In addition it can reduce fluid accumulation in the legs.

PRACTICE. Spread your mat and place a bolster lengthwise on it, with a folded blanket at the far end sufficient to support your head. Sit in Swastikasana (6.11b) in front of the bolster. Lean back onto your elbows. Exhale and lie back over the bolster, with your head supported by the blanket.

Release your shoulder blades away from your ears. Draw your breastbone toward your chin, and lift your chest. Broaden your breastbone and spread your collarbones. Use your hands to lengthen the back of your neck, so your throat softens. Place your arms on the floor and turn them out at their sockets (8.6a). Release the abdomen. Relax your hearing inward. Allow your breath to be soft and quiet.

Do not come up to change sides. Switch legs in the prone position, and repeat with the other leg on top. To come out, undo your legs. Bend your knees and place your feet on the floor. Turn to your side and sit up.

SUPTA SWASTIKASANA WITH BLANKETS. Place folded blankets under your knees to further relax your abdominal organs (8.6b)

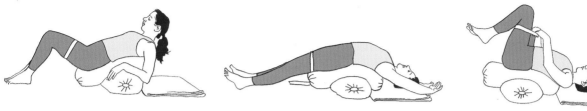

8.7B CURVE BACK 8.7C FINAL POSE 8.7D BEND KNEES, REMOVE STRAP

8.7

Viparita Dandasana I
Back Bend over Crossed Bolsters

BENEFITS. At once energizing and restful, this supported back bend can help you recover from the day's fatigue before you begin your yoga practice. It creates mobility in the spine, releases tension in the diaphragm, and allows the breath to deepen. The inner organs spread and lengthen, particularly the lungs and chest, which are at the apex of this version. Circulation is increased throughout the adrenal and thyroid glands. Depression and mood swings are counteracted (if you are depressed, practice with your eyes open), so this pose can help alleviate premenstrual tension.

PRACTICE. Place a bolster on the floor. Place another bolster across the center of the first to form a cross. Position one or more folded blankets on the floor, in line with the top bolster. Have a thinly rolled blanket at hand.

Sit slightly toward the foot end of the top bolster, with the blankets behind you, with your knees bent and feet on the floor. Secure the tops of your thighs with a strap (8.7a). Lie back with your spine aligned along the center of the bolster and elbows on the blanket (8.7b). Lie down all the way, allowing your shoulders to hang free, not touching the floor. Rest the top of the back of your head on the folded blanket. Slide the rolled blanket under your neck. Bend your arms out to the sides and rest them on the floor, slightly above your head. Stretch your legs and allow your feet to fall out to the sides (8.7c).

Feel the release as the chest takes on the shape of the support. Let the spine open evenly along its length. Observe yourself in the pose, the way a child would: innocently and without judgment. Experience each moment fully.

To come out, bend your knees and remove the strap (8.7d). Push the bolsters away from you and slide back (8.7e). Allow your lower back to settle on the floor for a few moments. Turn onto your side and push up.

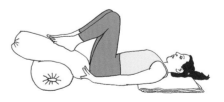

8.7E SLIDE BACK, REST LOWER BACK

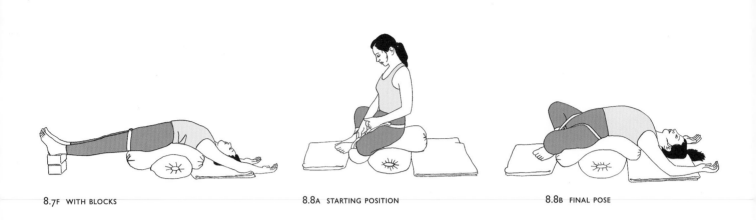

8.7F WITH BLOCKS   8.8A STARTING POSITION   8.8B FINAL POSE

CAUTIONS. Do not practice this pose if you have a migraine headache. Check that you are properly positioned over the bolsters: your head and shoulders should not be in Setu Banda Sarvangasana (8.9c), and your head should not be hanging off the end of the bolster with your neck crunched.

VIPARITA DANDASANA I WITH BLOCKS. If you experience lower back pain, support your feet on blocks (8.7f). If a backache persists, bend your knees and place your feet on the floor. Alternatively you can begin with a lower support, such as two rectangularly folded blankets that are crossed on top of each other.

8.8
Supta Baddha Konasana in Viparita Dandasana I
Bound-Angle Pose
over Crossed Bolsters

BENEFITS. As with the other versions of Supta Baddha Konasana, this one reduces abdominal cramps. It also relieves abdominal inflammation and is particularly effective when cramps or an excessive menstrual flow are caused by endometriosis. This variation circulates an abundance of blood and pranic energy around the reproductive organs.

PRACTICE. Place a bolster on the floor. Lay another bolster across the center of the first to form a cross. Place folded blankets on either end of the second bolster for your head, shoulders, and the feet to rest on. Adjust the number of blankets to decrease or increase the intensity of the back bend; more blankets give you less abdominal stretch. If the back bend causes lower back pain, support your shoulders and feet with more blankets. Keep in mind though that the greater the back arch and subsequent abdominal stretch, the more effective the pose will be in relieving abdominal spasms.

Sit on top of the top bolster. Secure your feet with a strap, as for Supta Baddha Konasana I (8.8a). Slide forward off the bolster a little, so the outer edges of your feet are close to the floor. Curve back over the bolster and rest the back of your head on the floor or folded blanket. Position your arms out to the sides (8.8b).

Allow the placement of the hips and lower back on the bolster to be determined by the location of your menstrual discomfort or pain. If cramping is caused by endometriosis, observe where the pain is at its most intense, and bring

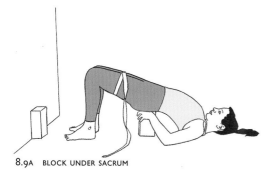

8.9A   BLOCK UNDER SACRUM

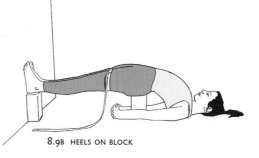

8.9B   HEELS ON BLOCK

maximum extension and opening to that area.

If you experience strain in your lower back, hold the ends of the bolster firmly and raise your hips off the bolster. Then lengthen the lumbar spine by firming the buttock muscles and sliding your tailbone toward your heels. Release your hips and lower spine back over the bolster.

To come out, raise your knees a little and slip your feet out of the strap. Slide the bolster away from you, and roll back down onto the floor, knees bent. Rest for a minute to allow your lower back to recover from the back bend. Turn over onto one side and push up with your hands.

CAUTIONS. If the stretch of the inner thighs causes pain, remove the strap and stretch your legs out in front of you, keeping your hips elevated on the bolster. If your lower back feels uncomfortable, come out of the pose, roll your knees over your chest, and hold your shins for 30 seconds.

8.9
Setu Bandha Sarvangasana I
Supported Bridge Pose with Blocks

BENEFITS. This pose is both revitalizing and calming. The chin lock pacifies the throat and helps calm a restless mind. It also helps balance the thyroid and the parathyroid glands by bathing them with an abundant supply of blood. The back-bending action tones the kidneys and adrenal glands and opens the chest, which helps to lift depression and relieve anxiety. Fluctuating blood pressure is stabilized, and migraines and insomnia are relieved.

This supported version of the classic pose improves posture. If you allow your upper spine to slouch forward, it will eventually become stiff and weak. Regular practice of this pose counteracts this tendency by creating flexibility in the upper spine and shoulder joints.

PRACTICE. Sit on your mat, facing the wall and a few feet away from it, with your knees slightly bent. Place an upright block against the wall and place a second block to one side. Secure the tops of your thighs with a strap.

Lie down, with your knees bent. Roll your shoulders back so your chest expands. Raise your pelvis as high as you can and slide the block, positioned vertically, under your sacrum (8.9a). Stretch your legs out one at a time and rest your heels on the second block (8.9b). Keep your feet together and your legs straight. Open the soles of your feet to the wall. Extend your arms along the floor toward your feet. Interlock your fingers behind

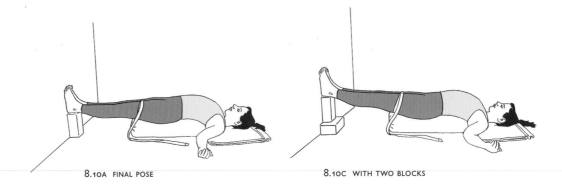

8.10A FINAL POSE

8.10C WITH TWO BLOCKS

the block and pull your wrists away from each other. Against the resistance of your arms, roll onto the very tops of your shoulders and coil your back ribs in. This action brings the breastbone closer to the chin and dynamically opens the chest. Then, without disturbing the lift of the upper back and chest, release your arms to the sides, slightly away from your trunk. Turn the upper arms out, so the palms face the ceiling (8.9c). Allow your breath to become quiet and even.

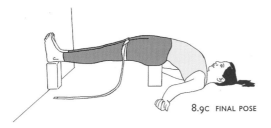

8.9C FINAL POSE

To come out, bend your knees and place your feet on the floor. Raise your pelvis, slide the block out from under you, and release your pelvis down to rest on the floor. Remove the strap. Roll onto your right side. Press your left hand to the floor and sit up, raising your head last.

CAUTIONS. It takes time for the body to become pliable. If you are a beginner or are stiff, practice Setu Banda Sarvangasana II rather than this pose until your upper back becomes more flexible.

8.10

Setu Bandha Sarvangasana II
Supported Bridge Pose with Bolster and Block

BENEFITS. Some women become emotionally vulnerable around the time of menstruation. Teenagers and those in perimenopause are particularly prone to depression and irritability at this time. In Setu Bandha Sarvangasana II, the supported expansion of the chest helps to stabilize emotions and defuse anxiety.

This pose gives you the opportunity to rest during menstruation. It quiets the brain, relieves diarrhea, and stabilizes the thyroid and parathyroid glands. Opening the chest enables the breath to flow more easily. You can practice it as a preparation for pranayama (see chapters 11 and 14) or as a resting pose at the end of a vigorous practice.

PRACTICE. Position the bolster on the floor, *not* on a mat, at a right angle to and approximately 1½ feet from the wall. The bolster should be located so that when you lie on it, the top edge of the bolster is at your lower rib area and your feet touch the wall. Place an upright block against the wall, in line with the middle of the bolster. Sit on the

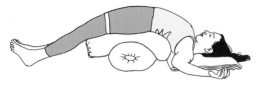

8.10D OVER CROSSED BOLSTERS

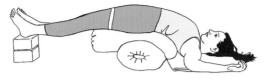

8.10E OVER CROOSED BOLSTERS, WITH BLOCKS

bolster, close to the wall. Secure the tops of your thighs with a strap (this will help keep the lower abdominal area soft). Curve your torso back over the bolster, placing the tops of your shoulders and the back of your head on the floor, so your chest opens. Position your heels on the block, and allow the bottoms of your feet to touch the wall. (If your knees are still bent, hold the sides of the bolster and straighten your legs, so the bolster slides a little away from the wall.)

Roll your shoulders back. With your hands, lengthen the back of your neck and allow your throat to recede and relax. Roll your upper arms out. Rest them on the floor, slightly away from the sides of your torso, palms facing the ceiling (8.10a). Allow the breath to be gentle and even.

To come out, bend your knees and place your feet on the floor, beside the bolster. Raise your pelvis and slide the bolster away from you. Lower your pelvis to the floor. Remove the strap. Cross your legs and place them on the bolster. Let your lower back settle toward the floor. Rest there for a few moments. Turn to your right side. Push your left hand to the floor and sit up, bringing your head up last.

CAUTIONS. Do not practice this pose if you have a herniated disk.

SETU BANDHA SARVANGASANA II WITH ROLLED WASHCLOTH. If you suffer from migraine headaches or if you have an overactive thyroid, raise your head a little by placing a rolled washcloth under it. The roll should begin at the occipital bone, located at the base of your skull. (8.10b).

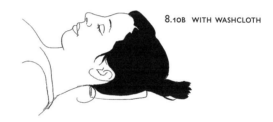

8.10B WITH WASHCLOTH

SETU BANDHA SARVANGASANA II WITH TWO BLOCKS. Lower back pain in this pose indicates stiffness in the upper back. With practice, poses such as this one create flexibility in the upper spine, and lower back pain dissipates. However, for some students, lower back pain in this pose is unbearable and this must be listened to! Raise your feet higher with a second block until you can practice pain free (8.10c). Over time, reduce the height of the support as your upper back becomes more flexible.

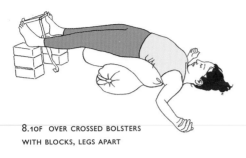

8.10F OVER CROSSED BOLSTERS
WITH BLOCKS, LEGS APART

SETU BANDHA SARVANGASANA II OVER CROSSED BOLSTERS. In this pose, the combination of the chin lock and the expanded chest has a very calming effect on the nerves and brain; thyroid function is balanced, the mind becomes quiet, and anxiety is reduced. Those with insomnia may therefore find that this variation, when practiced in combination with supported inverted poses (see chapter 18), will allow drowsiness to settle in. Set up the crossed bolsters, but this time sit a little farther up on the bolster. Place a strap around the middle of your thighs. Curve back over the bolster. Rest the back of your head and the *very tops* of your shoulders on the folded blankets. Release your arms to the sides and turn your upper arms out (8.10d). The abdomen now forms the apex of the pose, making this extremely effective in relieving menstrual cramps and reducing diarrhea. If you experience low back pain, practice this pose with the feet up on blocks (8.10e).

SETU BANDHA SARVANGASANA OVER CROSSED BOLSTERS WITH STRAP, BLOCKS, AND LEGS APART. This pose has a cooling effect on the uterus and helps to stem a heavy flow. If you are experiencing excessive bleeding, regardless of the reason, separate your legs approximately 3 feet apart, and support them on blocks, so your feet do not drop below the level of the pelvis. Tuck your tailbone toward your feet so your pubic bone aligns above it. Slip a looped strap around each big toe to prevent the feet and thighs from rolling out (8.10f). Observe how your abdominal organs relax and drop down into the pelvis.

8.11
Supta Baddha Konasana in Setu Bandhasana
Reclining Bound-Angle in Supported Bridge Pose

BENEFITS. The combination of these two poses decongests the pelvic organs. Circulation around the reproductive organs is increased, and tension and any sensation of pressure within the pelvis is released. This helps to alleviate any heaviness or inflammation there. It also relieves menstrual cramps and, with patient and persistent practice, helps reduce an excessive menstrual flow. Practice this pose at any time, not just during menstruation, to keep menstrual problems at bay and relieve anxiety.

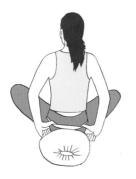

8.11A POSITION STRAP

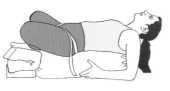

8.11B CURVE BACK

8.11C FINAL POSE

PRACTICE. Place a bolster on the floor (not on a mat) and a flat block on the foot end. Have a folded blanket and a strap to hand. Sit in the middle of the bolster. Bring the soles of your feet together on top of the block. Secure your feet with a strap, as described for Supta Baddha Konasana I (8.2b). Draw your heels up close to your groin and tighten the strap. Position the strap below the tailbone, to help align the tailbone directly below the pubic bone (8.11a). This will help you avoid pain in and maintain traction through the lumbar spine. In addition it will keep the abdomen free from strain.

Wedge the folded blanket between your feet and the block. Lean back onto your elbows. Raise your pelvis and tuck your tailbone toward your heels. Curve your upper back over the bolster, placing the very tops of your shoulders and the back of your head on the floor (8.11b). Turn your upper arms out, so the palms face the ceiling (8.11c). Let your knees and thighs release to the sides and your belly to soften. Relax your eyes and throat.

Allow the muscles on either side of the spine to flow over the sides of the bolster. The uterus is drawn down to the back of the pelvis and is rested. Relax your facial muscles, your eyes, and your throat. Make a fist with your hands; then allow the fingers to release from the grip. Remain quietly in this pose for as long as you can, without resistance or distraction. Keep the breath soft and relaxed.

To come out, slip your feet out of the strap. Place your feet on the floor, on either side of the bolster. Raise your hips off the bolster, inhale, and slide it away from you. Rest your pelvis on the floor. Cross your legs and place them on the bolster. Wait for a few moments for the lower back to settle. Turn to your side and sit up.

CAUTIONS. Do not practice this pose if you have a herniated disk or experience inner groin pain. If you experience inner groin or lower back pain, remove the strap and stretch your legs out. Then practice Setu Bandha Sarvangasana I instead (8.9c).

SUPTA BADDHA KONASANA IN SETU BANDHASANA WITH ROLLED WASHCLOTH. To pacify an overactive thyroid (hyperthyroidism), raise your head with a rolled washcloth, as described in Setu Banda Sarvangasana II with Rolled Washcloth (8.10b.)

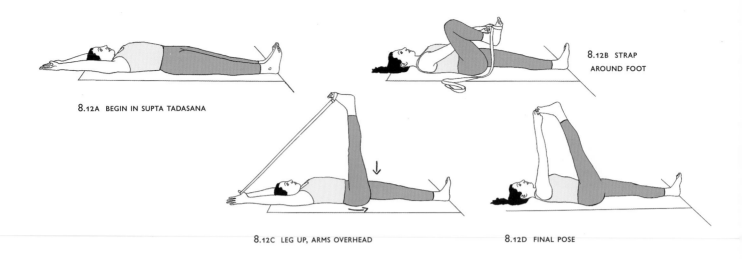

8.12A BEGIN IN SUPTA TADASANA

8.12B STRAP AROUND FOOT

8.12C LEG UP, ARMS OVERHEAD

8.12D FINAL POSE

8.12

Supta Padangustasana I
Reclining Big-Toe Pose

BENEFITS. This pose releases the hamstrings, creates movement and freedom through the pelvic joints, and reduces fluid accumulation in the legs. It also incorporates a stretch through the shoulders and breasts.

PRACTICE. In all poses, women should take care not to harden the belly. Do not to initiate this hamstring work from the abdomen. Keep the belly soft and relaxed throughout.

Place the short end of your mat against the wall. Lie on the mat with your chest, hips, and feet aligned. Spread the soles of your feet and place them against the wall. Inhale, raise your arms above your head, and hook your thumbs together (8.12a). Stretch out into your fingertips and press your thighs to the floor. Change the hook of your thumbs and repeat.

Make a small loop at the end of the strap. Bend your right knee and hook the strap around the ball of your right foot (8.12b). Take hold of the loop with your right hand. Simultaneously raise your leg to a right angle and straighten it, then

slide your hands to the end of the strap until your arms are stretched over your head (8.12c).

Work on the alignment of the pelvis and torso: both sides of the trunk should be equal in length. Rotate your left leg in, so your foot points straight up. Press your left thighbone down. Press your right upper thigh away from you and also down onto the right sacral joint. Lengthen the right side of your pelvis through your right buttock bone.

When you can do the pose with the pelvis straight, that is, without the right hip tilting toward you and without the legs bending, take hold of your big toe with your first two fingers and thumb, and draw your upper leg toward your head (8.12d). To come out, bend your right knee, release the strap, and rest your leg on the floor. Repeat on the other side.

CAUTIONS. Avoid this pose during menstruation, as the weight of the lifted leg bearing down on the uterus presents a strain.

Some women have flexible hamstrings and can easily pull their leg over their head. If you are a beginner, do not draw your leg toward your head until you have built strength in the legs and understand how to work with alignment. To avoid overstretching the ligaments and weakening the hip joints, keep the lifted leg vertical, at a right angle to the floor.

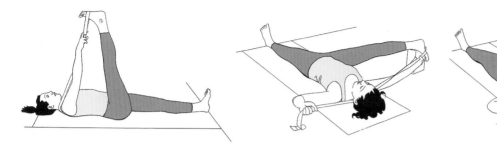

8.13A HOLD LOOPED STRAP   8.13B FINAL POSE   8.13C WITH BOLSTER

8.13

Supta Padangustasana II
Reclining Big-Toe Pose to the Side

BENEFITS. It is important for women to practice this pose regularly, because it helps keep the reproductive organs healthy. With regular practice, flexibility in the hip joints and correct alignment of the hip joints can be achieved more readily. This work helps counteract abdominal tension and the development of uterine fibroids and other diseases of the abdominal organs. It also strengthens the pelvic muscles, tones the internal organs, and creates elasticity in the hamstrings and inner thighs.

PRACTICE. Come into Supta Padangusthasana I with a strap around your foot (8.12b). If you can hold your leg up at a right angle and without hardening the belly or overarching the lumbar spine, you can continue with Supta Padangustasana II. (If you cannot, then practice with Supta Padangusthasana I.)

Make the loop of the strap bigger. Slip the first two fingers of your right hand through the loop (8.13a). Pass the other end of the strap behind your neck and let it rest on the floor. Press your left thigh and shinbone down. Open the soles of the left foot and keep the ball of your foot pressed against the wall. Exhale and swing your right leg out to the right. Place your foot on the block. Brace your right elbow and upper arm on the floor. Hold the end of the strap with your left hand and, with a pulley action, draw your foot toward your shoulder (8.13b).

Firm your knees and thighs and stretch and open the backs of both knees. To prevent yourself from tipping to the right and to facilitate a stretch across the pelvis and upper torso, anchor your left shoulder, rib cage, and pelvis into the floor. Extend from your inner right groin out to your inner right anklebone. Draw the back of your right thigh in toward your right hip socket.

Roll both shoulders away from your ears and hook your shoulder blades sharply into your upper back. Lift and broaden the chest, and spread the collarbones. Keep the back of your neck long and your chin slightly lower than your forehead. Breathe evenly and naturally. As always, avoid overarching the lumbar spine, because this can strain the pelvic organs.

To come out, return your leg to Supta Padangustasana I. Bend your leg, remove the strap, and place your leg on the floor. Repeat on the other side. Turn to one side and come up, quietly maintaining your sense of well-being.

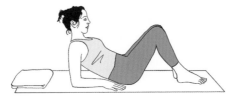

8.14A LIE BACK   8.14B POSITION BLANKET

CAUTIONS. Avoid this pose if you have a groin pull.

SUPTA PADANGUSTASANA II WITH BOLSTER. If you are experiencing menstrual difficulties, such as a heavy flow, abdominal cramps, or tiredness, or if you have inner knee pain, place a bolster under the thigh of the diagonal leg (8.13c). Do not try to go to your limit, but rest in the pose, so there is no strain or tension and the abdominal muscles remain soft.

8.14
Savasana
Relaxation Pose

BENEFITS. Also known as Corpse Pose, Savasana frees the body from tension and recharges the batteries. When the muscles and joints are consciously relaxed, the nerves are soothed and the mind becomes quiet. With regular practice, we learn to draw our awareness in and away from external events and stimuli, setting the mind at ease. Do this pose at the end of your practice or any time you feel you would benefit from spending a few quiet moments.

PRACTICE. Have one blanket nearby to place under your head. Dim the lights. Sit on the floor on your mat, with your legs bent and your feet flat on the floor. The center of your chest, your pelvis, and your inner legs and heels should be aligned. Lean back onto your elbows and lower your spine to the floor (8.14a). Place the folded blanket so that it supports your head and neck (8.14b).

Stretch your legs out, one at a time, extending from the backs of the thighs to the heels (8.14c). Let your feet fall out to the sides and relax them completely. Take care to keep the weight even on both sides of your pelvis and legs; we get dragged back into our thoughts if the body is tilted to one side.

Do not allow your head to tip back or roll to the side. With your hands, readjust your head so it rests exactly on the center of the back of the skull. Gently lengthen the back of the skull away from your neck. Relax your throat.

Roll your shoulders away from your ears. Spread your shoulder blades to the sides and allow them to rest flat on the floor. Open your arms comfortably out to the sides so there is space between your upper arms and your chest. Rotate your upper arms out at their sockets; let your

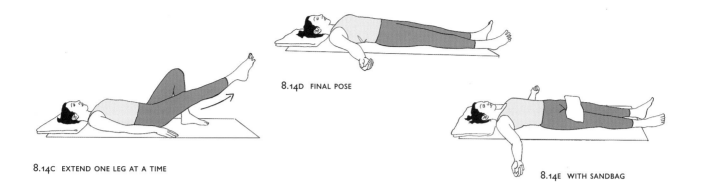

8.14C EXTEND ONE LEG AT A TIME

8.14D FINAL POSE

8.14E WITH SANDBAG

palms face the ceiling and relax your hands. Close your eyes (8.14d).

Having placed yourself carefully, the rest of the pose is practiced without moving the physical body. Allow your joints to loosen and your bones, even those of the skull, to release. Feel your body supported by the floor.

Release any tension in the soles of the feet and ankles. Allow the deep muscles of the calves to feel like liquid. Relax the pelvis and genitals, inside and out. Feel the vast, deep, and serene space in the groins and belly as the pelvic organs relax.

Allow your spine to release along its length. Allow the muscles of the arms and shoulders to fall away from the bones.

Release the skin on the forehead, from the hairline to the eyebrows. Feel the softness of the scalp and allow it to become loose. Release all the tiny muscles around the eyes. Make space between the eyebrows and allow your brow to spread outward. Withdraw your gaze from the outer world, and look inward and down toward your navel.

Relax your inner ears inward. Relax the back of the nostrils. Let go of your lower jaw, so your upper teeth and lower teeth are not clenched together. Allow your teeth to be cradled by your

gums, and lengthen them away from your nose. A hyperactive tongue indicates unspoken words and a hyperactive heart. Relax the tongue and let it rest it lightly on your lower palate. Let go completely, so there is no energy flowing out of you, only energy flowing in.

As you move deeper into the pose, have a sense of the pores of the skin over the entire body drawing inward. As the mind and body become still, the breath becomes shallow and quiet. Rest in the peacefulness within.

So the stillness of the pose is not disturbed, take your time before you engage with the world. When you feel you are ready, inhale and exhale deeply. Bend your arms and legs. Turn onto your right side and draw your knees toward your chest. Cradle your head in the crook of your elbow or rest it on a blanket. Draw your energies in toward your womb and wait for a few moments. Then draw your head toward your knees and, bowing to your inner self, sit up gently, pushing up and away from your hands. Raise your head last.

CAUTIONS. If you are very upset or traumatized by some external event, practice with your eyes open.

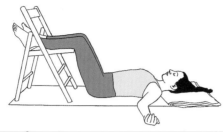

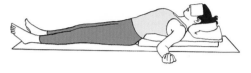

8.14F WITH LEGS SUPPORTED ON CHAIR   8.14G WITH UPPER BACK SUPPORTED

SAVASANA WITH HEAD WRAP. Savasana can be done with a head wrap or a small towel placed over the eyes (8.1c).

SAVASANA WITH SANDBAG. To settle the nervous system and release body tension, place a sandbag across the tops of your thighs (8.14e). This also works wonderfully to reduce lower back pain during menstruation.

SAVASANA WITH LEGS SUPPORTED ON CHAIR. Rest with your calves supported on a chair seat (8.14f). You can practice this variation during your period to prevent blood pooling in the abdomen, but make sure your legs are not folded up too close to your torso. You can practice it to rest the heart, relieve abdominal tension and lower back pain, or at the end of a back bend practice or supported inversions sequence—for example, after Salambha Sarvangasana I (9.3f), followed by Ardha Halasana (9.6b).

SAVASANA WITH UPPER BACK SUPPORTED. Opening the chest relaxes and opens the lungs and intercostals, which prepares them for breathing. When pranayama is practiced reclining over a support (all the pranayama exercises in this book are practiced this way), space is created for the lungs, which allows breathing to be deeper and easier.

In addition the expansion of the chest cavity in this pose makes it an effective way to relax for those who are prone to depression or who suffer from asthma. Some of my women students report a marked increase in asthma attacks during the premenstrual phase of their cycle.

Fold two blankets into a narrow rectangular shape and on top of each other. Place them along the center of your mat and at the top end.

Sit on your mat, facing away from your blankets. Position yourself over them, so they support you from your lower back to your head. Come into Savasana with Upper Back Supported (8.14g). A woman's intercostals muscles, located under the breasts, have less elasticity than a man's. Consequently she has to make more of an effort to lengthen the rib cage and roll the tops of the shoulders back. Slide your shoulder blades down your back and tuck the bottom of your shoulder blades into your chest, so that the chest lifts. Raise your front ribs, *but not your shoulders*, up toward your head, so the area under the breasts has some freedom. Turn your upper arms out at the shoulder joints. Allow the rib cage to expand over the support. Let the belly relax and spread to the sides. Surrender the intelligence of the brain to the wisdom of the heart, and listen for your own inner vibration.

9

Inverted Poses: Balancing the System

WE SPEND MUCH of our time in an upright position: standing, walking, sitting. Whenever we are upright, gravity exerts a downward pull on our bodies, which contributes to the aging process. To some extent, we can reverse this process by practicing inversions: yoga poses in which we turn ourselves upside down. Inversions promote good health and longevity. For mental tiredness, go upside down and refresh your brain. For nervous exhaustion, invert your body to calm the nerves and sleep more soundly. The inversions revitalize the organs, fortify the digestive system, keep the bowels regular, and boost the immune system. Additionally the legs are given a complete rest, and varicose veins are kept at bay.

Many women today rely on makeup and surgery to maintain a youthful appearance. Yoga offers a more fundamental and integrated beauty regime—inverted poses. They increase blood flow to the face and neck, arresting the physical signs of aging and dramatically improving appearance. The woman who regularly practices inversions has eyes that shine, glossy hair, and a bloom in her cheeks.

But perhaps the most profound effect of these poses on women occurs via the endocrine system. The health and stability of the hormonal cycle throughout the month depends on the balanced interaction of various endocrine glands with each other and with the nervous system. Through the practice of inversions, the blood is encouraged to flow around the major glands in the head and neck, irrigating them with nourishment. These changes in the circulation help to regulate hormone balance by more efficiently transporting hormonal "messages" around the body. The reproductive system is thus strengthened and menstrual problems are kept at bay.

General Cautions for Practicing Inverted Poses

When practicing the inverted poses presented in this chapter, remember to follow these guidelines. Cautions are also included with each pose.

- Do not practice the inverted poses if you are menstruating or if you have neck injuries, detached retina, or a sinus or ear infection.

- If you have any type of headache, wait until it passes before practicing the inversions.

- Do not practice the inverted poses if you have diarrhea or if you feel nauseous before or during the pose.

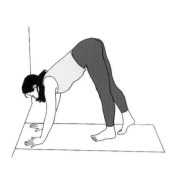 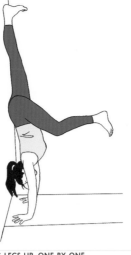 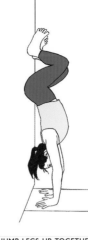

9.1A STARTING POSITION   9.1B SWING LEGS UP, ONE BY ONE   9.1C JUMP LEGS UP TOGETHER   9.1D FINAL POSE

9.1

Adho Mukha Vrksasana
Arm Balance

BENEFITS. In Sanskrit, Adho Mukha Vrksasana literally means Downward-Facing Tree Pose. Often called Arm Balance, this pose is an important counterbalance to the standing poses. This inverted, weight-bearing posture strengthens the shoulders, arms, and wrists and brings energy and vitality to the whole body.

PRACTICE. Spread your mat with the short end touching the wall. Facing the wall, reach down and place your hands on the floor, two to three inches away from the wall and shoulder-width apart (9.1a). Spread your fingers and press your hands down. (If you have weak wrists, support the heels of your hands on a folded nonslip mat.) Straighten your arms and legs, swing your pelvis closer to the wall, and lift through your sitting bones. Draw your shoulder blades away from

your neck and move them deep into your upper back.

With an exhalation, swing one leg up and quickly follow it with the second leg. Rest your heels against the wall (9.1b). In the beginning, jump with whichever leg takes you up the easiest. Later on, learn to jump with the other leg, and then with both legs together (9.1c). Don't be discouraged if you don't get up the first time. This beginning movement is in itself energizing, and by practicing it regularly and repeatedly you will eventually get up into the pose.

Once up, press down through the knuckles at the base of the fingers, squeeze your elbows toward each other, pull up from your elbow joints, and slide your heels farther up the wall. Spread your collarbones. Move your shoulders away from the wall, and move your elbows toward the wall. Firm your buttock muscles and pull your tailbone and sacrum up. Draw your kneecaps into your legs and rotate your thighs in (9.1d). Relax your head and neck. Breathe! Do not let your lumbar sink (9.1e, incorrect pose).

To come out, continue lifting up through your

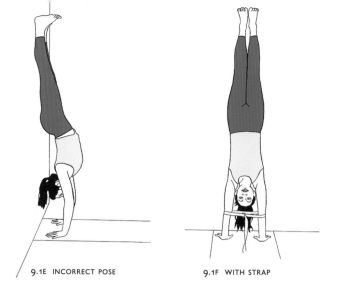

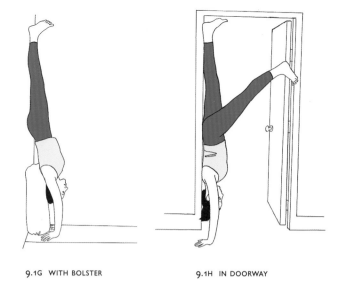

9.1E INCORRECT POSE   9.1F WITH STRAP   9.1G WITH BOLSTER   9.1H IN DOORWAY

shoulders and hips. With straight arms, come down one leg at a time.

CAUTIONS. Do not practice this pose if you have carpal tunnel syndrome or if you cannot support your weight on your arms.

ADHO MUKHA VRKSASANA WITH STRAP. If you cannot straighten your arms, place a strap around them: if you are bending at the forearms, place it just below the elbows; if you are bending at the upper arms, place it just above the elbows (9.1f).

ADHO MUKHA VRKSASANA WITH BOLSTER. If you are having difficulty getting up in the pose, place an upright bolster on the mat, against the wall. As you kick up, allow your head to push against the bolster. Against this resistance, you will find it easier to learn the mechanics of getting up into the pose (9.1g). When this becomes easy, go up without the bolster.

ADHO MUKHA VRKSASANA IN DOORWAY. If you are new to this pose, if you cannot kick up into the pose, or if your arms are weak, work in a doorway. (You will need a wide doorframe, such as a front door.) This modification will familiarize you with the inverted position and will strengthen your arms and wrists in preparation for practicing against the wall.

Face the nondoor side the doorframe, reach down and place your palms on the floor, at either side of the frame and shoulder-width apart. Point your middle finger straight ahead. Press your hands down, straighten your arms, and lift your pelvis. Support your back against the frame.

Walk your feet as high as you can up the opposite side of the doorframe. Avoid the door itself though, because it may move if you put your feet on it. Lift your shoulders. Draw your tailbone up and away from the back of your waist. Fully stretch your legs (9.1h). To come out, walk back down the doorframe with your arms straight.

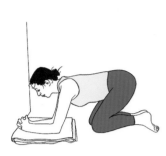

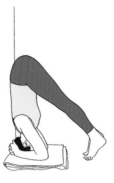

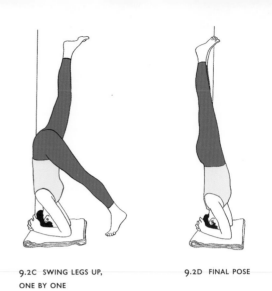

9.2A STARTING POSITION   9.2B LIFT HIPS   9.2C SWING LEGS UP, ONE BY ONE   9.2D FINAL POSE

9.2

Salamba Sirsasana
Headstand

BENEFITS. Salamba Sirsasana offers many wide-ranging benefits. Known as the Father of Asanas, this pose invigorates the entire being, but its primary benefit is that it refreshes the circulation of blood to the brain and master glands—the pituitary, the pineal, and the hypothalamus. It provides an oxygen wash to the head, which counteracts tiredness, improves concentration, and increases intellectual capacity. Headstand improves the functioning of the sense organs, too. It can, for example, improve eyesight. It strengthens respiration, increases circulation, and helps bring the uterus into proper position. Regular practice will help you to develop self-confidence, willpower, and emotional stability. Together with Salamba Sarvangasana I (9.3f), Halasana (9.6b), and Setu Bandha Sarvangasana with Chair (9.3m), Salamba Sirsasana (9.2d) helps to keep the menstrual cycle balanced and healthy.

PRACTICE. Practice Salamba Sirsasana against the wall until you have developed the strength and balance required to keep you steady and safe in the pose. Fold your mat into four and place it against the wall. Position a blanket (folded to the width of your mat) on top of the mat for extra padding. Kneel down facing the wall.

Place your elbows on the blanket, forearm-distance apart. Interlace your fingers, and place the outer edges of your cupped hands on the mat, with your knuckles lightly touching to the wall. Keep your hands perpendicular to the floor and your elbows directly beneath your shoulders (9.2a).

Place your head on the mat, making sure that the back of your head is in contact with your hands and that you are centered on the crown of your head. (Do not balance toward the back of the head, as it strains the cervical spine and neck muscles.) Firmly press your outer wrist bones and forearms into the floor. Lift your shoulders away from the floor. Straighten your legs and raise your hips. Walk your feet toward your head. Be on the tips of your toes, and fully stretch the back of your knees. Lift your hips and curve them toward the wall, but avoid touching your upper back to the wall (9.2b).

Spread your shoulder blades away from each other and move them deep into your upper back. Swing your legs up, one at a time (9.2c), and place your feet against the wall (9.2d). (As you gain in strength and confidence, practice away from the

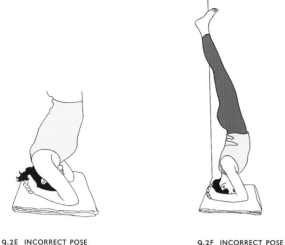

9.2E INCORRECT POSE

9.2F INCORRECT POSE

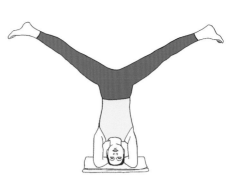

9.2G UPAVISTHA KONASANA IN SALAMBA SIRSASANA

wall, a few inches at a time, until you can balance unsupported.)

A successful Salamba Sirsasana depends on two things: the skill with which you can lift your body up and away from your neck and shoulders and the correct alignment of the spine. If the lumbar spine is allowed to sink forward into the abdominal area, pressure is brought to bear on the uterus and ovaries, which may create hardness and tension there (9.2e, incorrect pose).

Lift your lumbar spine, firm your buttock muscles, and draw your tailbone in toward your pubic bone and up toward your feet. Lift up from the backs of your knees to avoid a banana-shaped pose (9.2f, incorrect pose). Rotate your thighs toward each other.

To complete the pose, pull up from your inner shins and join your feet together. Extend up through your inner heels and the inner balls of your feet and flex your toes toward you. As with all the inverted postures, the legs should feel full and strong.

With regular practice, Salamba Sirsasana becomes stable and light. When the balance is even on the left and right sides of the body, including the skull, the mind becomes quiet and centered.

If you are practicing at the wall, keep your shoulder blades lifted and firmly pressed into your back ribs, and come down with bent legs.

If you are away from the wall, and you can do so without collapsing your upper back, come down with straight legs.

CAUTIONS. Do not practice Salamba Sirsasana if you have a shoulder or neck injury, high blood pressure, or a migraine headache. Do not practice Salamba Sirsasana if you are menstruating; wait until the flow has completely stopped. Similarly, if menstruation appears to have come to an end but bleeding resumes within one hour of practicing Salamba Sirsasana, menstruation has not finished. Wait until the flow has completely ceased. If your menstrual flow has ceased but resumes 5 hours after you practice Salamba Sirsasana, this is most likely the final expulsion of blood.

Always counterbalance Salamba Sirsasana with Salamba Sarvangasana (9.3f). When practiced together, these poses harmonize the glandular system and bring about a wonderful combination of mental clarity and mental calmness. If Salamba Sirsasana is practiced casually, you may compress your neck; beginners are strongly advised to learn this pose with the help of a competent teacher.

UPAVISTHA KONASANA IN SALAMBA SIRSASANA. This variation stretches and exercises the pelvic floor, pelvic organs, and groins. It provides the reproductive organs, internal and external, with

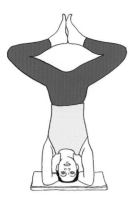

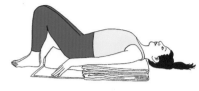

9.2H BADDHA KONASANA
IN SALAMBA SIRSASANA

9.3A STARTING POSITION

a fresh supply of blood. It also helps correct a displaced or prolapsed uterus. When practiced for the three days following menstruation, this posture helps the uterus recover from the stress of menstruation. Because the pose takes some of the weight off the shoulders, you may be able to hold your Salamba Sirsasana for a little longer.

From Salamba Sirsasana, spread your legs wide apart and extend them through your inner ankles (9.2g). Face your toes out to the sides and activate them so the toes spread. Continue lifting your shoulders and draw your shoulder blades into your back. Align the pelvis, so the front and back of the pelvis are drawn into an upright position. Lift the sacrum and move the tailbone in. When finished, move into the next variation, Baddha Konasana in Salamba Sirsasana (9.2h).

BADDHA KONASANA IN SALAMBA SIRSASANA. This variation boosts the circulation in the pelvis and exercises and refreshes the pelvic organs and genitals. It relieves cystitis and constipation and re-duces leukorrhea. The pose also relaxes the uterus and aids its recovery after menstruation. It helps to correct a displaced or prolapsed uterus and prevent the formation of fibroids. There is less pressure on the shoulders in this variation. Practice this pose and Upavistha Konasana in Sirsasana as a rest stop during your Salamba Sirsasana, so you can stay up a little longer.

Maintaining the extension from your inner groins to your knees and keeping your tailbone tucked into your pelvis, bend your knees and bring the soles of your feet together (9.2h). Take care not to allow the lumbar spine to collapse into the belly or your chest to collapse into the upper back. Lift your sacrum. Firm your buttock muscles without hardening your abdomen. Spread the groins and move your inner thighs and knees away from each other. Press your feet together. Draw your heels into a position directly above the perineum. Return your legs to the center and return to Salamba Sirsasana.

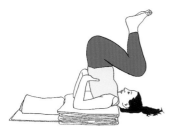

9.3B SWING HIPS UP

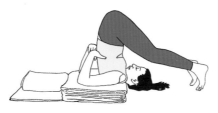

9.3C TOES ON FLOOR,
BEHIND HEAD

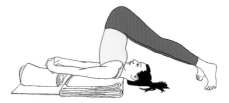

9.3D ROLL SHOULDERS UNDER,
STRETCH ARMS AWAY

9·3
Salamba Sarvangasana I
Supported Shoulderstand

BENEFITS. Salamba Sarvangasana I bestows a gentle energy to those who practice it. Known as the Mother of Asanas, it takes care of our health and brings forth those aspects of our nature that are patient and quiet.

The practice of Salamba Sarvangasana I increases the blood supply to the throat and chest. This nourishes and balances the thyroid and parathyroid glands as well as relieving problems in the nose, throat, and chest. Additionally it helps correct a displaced or prolapsed uterus, regulates blood pressure, and keeps menstrual dysfunction at bay. It helps the body eliminate toxins. When combined with its variations and the other inversions, as well as with the forward bends, it relieves constipation. Salamba Sarvangasana I soothes the nerves and brings about emotional stability. After practicing it, even for only a few minutes, you will feel refreshed and peaceful.

PRACTICE. In *The Woman's Yoga Book,* we will use Halasana (9.6b) to go into and come out of Salamba Sarvangasana I. Fold your mat into quar-

ters. Fold three blankets, individually, to the width of your mat. Stack them neatly, with folded edges lined up. Place the blanket stack on top of the mat. These supports are important; they protect the neck and prevent the chin from jamming into the chest. They also facilitate a stronger lift in the upper back than otherwise would be achieved on a flat surface.

Place a thickly folded blanket against the foot end of the blankets. This will make it easier for you to swing up into the pose. It will also soften your landing when you come down. Sit on the thickly folded blanket and lie back over the blankets, with your shoulders 2 to 3 inches away from the folded edge. Rest the back of your head on the floor. Place your arms by your sides with the palms facing the floor (9.3a).

Firm your upper arms against the blankets and slide your shoulder blades away from your neck. Bend your knees up over your chest. Then bend your elbows and, supporting your back with your hands, inhale and swing your hips up until your torso is perpendicular to the floor (9.3b) Place your toes on the floor behind your head and slowly straighten your legs (9.3c).

Come onto the tops of your shoulders. Interlace your fingers with your palms facing in, and stretch your arms away from your head (9.3d). Roll your upper arms and shoulders under you

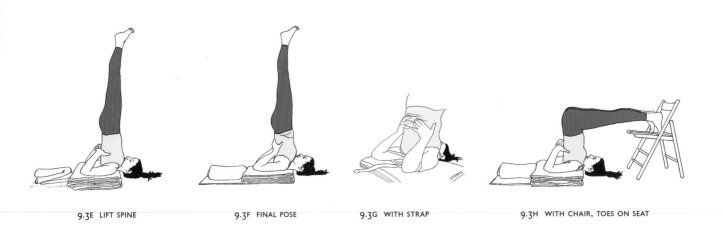

9.3E LIFT SPINE   9.3F FINAL POSE   9.3G WITH STRAP   9.3H WITH CHAIR, TOES ON SEAT

by rolling to the left and tucking your right shoulder under, then rolling to the right and tucking your left shoulder under. Press your outer upper arms into the floor. Change the interlock of the hands and repeat. Once again, place your hands on your back. Create length through the pelvis by lifting up through your inner groins and sit bones, so that your abdomen and chest are not compressed.

Now come into Salamba Sarvangasana I: if you are a beginning student, raise your legs, one at a time, and bring your body, from your shoulders to your heels, to vertical. As your practice progresses, you can hop your legs up from the floor with bent legs. Eventually, when your back is straight and strong, you can come up with straight legs.

Maintaining a dynamic lift through your torso and legs prevents this pose from becoming dull: press your upper arms down and use your hands to lift your spine (9.3e). Move your tailbone into your pelvis and balance the pelvis directly over the shoulders. Roll your thighs toward each other and extend up through the inner ankles (9.3f).

Women tend to have more hip and thigh weight than men. Consequently the lumbar spine may be the first thing to tire in Salamba Sarvangasana I. To avoid an aching back, move your hands even farther down your back toward the

shoulder blades and lift your spine higher. Extend through your inner ankles until your lumbar spine lengthens. This action strengthens and tones the abdominal organs. Practice with quiet eyes (don't stare at the ceiling) and a relaxed throat. To come down, return your legs to Halasana (9.6b). If you are a beginner, return one leg at a time.

CAUTIONS. Do not practice this pose or its variations if you are menstruating, have any back or neck injuries, or if you have diarrhea. Those with high blood pressure should practice Ardha Halasana (9.8d) for 3 to 10 minutes before attempting this pose. If you suffering from a migraine or tension headache, do not practice this pose until it has passed.

SALAMBA SARVANGASANA I WITH STRAP. When you are familiar with Salamba Sarvangasana I, you can practice it with a strap around your arms. This helps align your elbows with your shoulders, which enables you to lift your back with more strength.

Cinch the strap to form a loop that is the width of your shoulders. Sit on your blanket stack and slip one arm through the strap, so it rests just above your elbow. Lie down over both your blanket stack and the loose end of the strap. Raise your upper back and pelvis off the floor, and slip

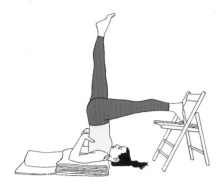
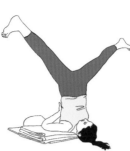
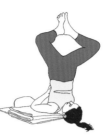
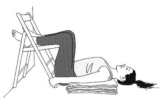

9.3I WITH CHAIR,
LIFTING ONE LEG AT A TIME

9.3J UPAVISTHA KONASANA
IN SALAMBA SARVANGASANA I

9.3K BADDHA KONASANA
IN SALAMBA SARVANGASANA I

9.3L SETU BANDHA SARVANGASANA
WITH CHAIR: STARTING POSITION

the strap around the other arm. Swing up into Halasana (9.6b) and then Salamba Sarvangasana I with Strap, as described (9.3g).

SALAMBA SARVANGASANA I WITH CHAIR. If you are a beginner, place a chair at leg length from and facing the folded edges of the blankets and place the tops of your toes on the chair seat (9.3h). Come up one leg at a time (9.3i). Your shoulders should be 1 inch in from the edge of the blankets. If you are sliding off the edge of the blankets, take a deep breath and come down. Start again with the shoulders a little farther in from the folded edge of the blankets.

UPAVISTA KONASANA IN SALAMBA SARVANGASANA I. This pose relaxes the uterus and helps it recover from the rigors of menstruation. It also brings flexibility to the hip joints. From Salamba Sarvangasana I, spread the legs wide and fully straighten them; pull up your knee caps and press out through your heels and the balls of your feet. Turn your toes out to the sides and flex them toward you. Bring your pelvis to an upright position: lift your sacrum and move your tailbone into your pelvis (9.3j).

BADDHA KONASANA IN SALAMBA SARVANGASANA I. This pose relaxes the uterus, reduces stiffness in

the pelvic joints, and helps relieve constipation. From Upavista Konasana in Salamba Sarvangasana I, bend your knees and bring the soles of your feet together. Lift your sacrum and tuck your tailbone into your pelvis so the pelvis is brought to an upright position. Press your feet together and your knees away from each other (9.3k). To come out, stretch your legs up and return to Salamba Sarvangasana I.

SETU BANDHA SARVANGASANA WITH CHAIR. This pose stimulates the adrenal glands, which in turn stimulate other glands to increased hormone production. It also benefits those with endometriosis, as it boosts circulation within the pelvic cavity and improves the function of the immune system.

Stack three or more blankets, folded to the dimensions of a four-fold mat. Position a chair with its back against the wall. Place your blanket stack on the floor, about 4 inches from the chair legs, with the folded edges facing into the room. Lie down on the blankets, with your shoulders a few inches from the folded edges and your legs on the chair seat (9.3l). Clasp the front legs of the chair with your hands. Brace your feet against the sides of the chair, inhale, and raise your pelvis off the floor. Walk your feet toward you and place your heels against the edge of the seat. Keep your thighs parallel. Lift one shoulder, roll it under, and

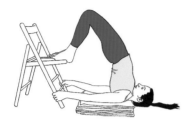

9.3M SETU BANDHA SARVANGASANA
WITH CHAIR: FINAL POSE

9.3N SETU BANDHA SARVANGASANA
WITH CHAIR: COMING DOWN

place it on the blanket. You should be on the top of that shoulder. Now do the same with the other shoulder.

Press your upper arms down and raise your pelvis higher. Firmly move your shoulder blades into your back until your back ribs are vertical, your chest expands, and your breastbone comes closer to your chin. Move the back of your thighs toward your buttocks, spread your toes, press your feet against the edge of the chair, and lift!

Feel your front body opening and stretching, as it receives the support and dynamic movement of the spine curving deeper into your back (9.3m).

To come out, release your grasp of the chair legs. Lower your pelvis to the floor and allow your feet to slide to the back of the chair. Lie with your back flat on the blankets and your lower legs resting on the chair for a few minutes (9.3n). Roll to your right side and come up.

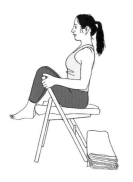

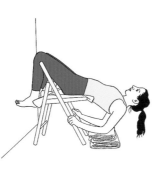

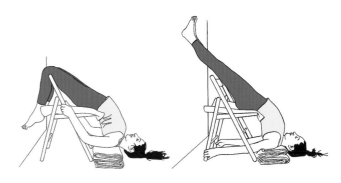

9.4A STARTING POSITION   9.4B CURVE BACK OVER CHAIR   9.4C SHOULDERS ON SUPPORT   9.4D BACK OF PELVIS SUPPORTED

9.4

Salamba Sarvangasana II
Supported Shoulderstand

BENEFITS. Very little muscular effort is involved in this version of Salamba Sarvangasana. Practice this at times when your energy is low, such as during the premenstrual phase. If you are a beginning student, the support will enable you to stay longer in the pose. It will also allow you to focus on pressing the shoulder blades into the back, which opens the chest, boosting circulation and allowing prana to flow abundantly around the breasts. In addition this pose draws the internal pelvic organs away from the pelvic floor and toward the spine, which helps relieve inflammation or pressure in the lower abdomen. Salamba Sarvangasana II helps the body heal after surgery or a major illness.

PRACTICE. Place a chair about two feet away from the wall, facing into the room. Position your narrowly folded blankets at the foot of the chair, with the folded edges facing away from the chair. Place a folded mat on the chair seat, to cover the front edge.

Sit astride the chair, facing the wall. Hold the sides of the chair and hook your knees, one by one, over the chair back (9.4a). Slide your hands down the front legs of the chair as you slowly curve back over the chair seat (9.4b). Gently release the tops of your shoulders onto the support (9.4c). Rest the *back* of your head (not the top) on the floor. Thread you hands through the chair and take hold of its back legs. Straighten your legs, one at a time. Rest your heels against the wall, with the inner edges of your feet together. The back of your pelvis is supported against the chair seat (9.4d).

Lift and firm your back ribs, and draw your breastbone closer to your chin. Roll your shoulders underneath you. Open your chest. If you feel secure, release your arms and rest them out to the sides (9.4e). Otherwise, continue to hold the back legs.

If you are continuing on with the variations, do not come out of the pose. To come out, bend your knees and place your feet on the back of the chair. Slide your buttocks off the chair and bring them to rest on the folded blankets. Support your calves on the chair seat. Rest for a few moments. Allow your lower back to drop toward the floor and your belly to relax. Turn to the side and push up from your hands.

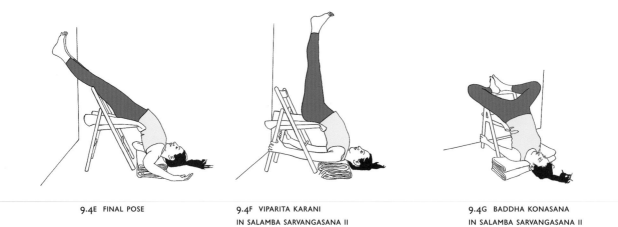

9.4E FINAL POSE

9.4F VIPARITA KARANI
IN SALAMBA SARVANGASANA II

9.4G BADDHA KONASANA
IN SALAMBA SARVANGASANA II

CAUTIONS. If you are a beginning student, ask your teacher to take you into this pose until you have the confidence and skill to come into it by yourself. Do not practice during menstruation or if you are suffering from any kind of headache. If you slide off the blankets while in the pose, come down, take a deep breath, and start again.

VIPARITA KARANI IN SALAMBA SARVANGASANA II. This version provides the potential for a tremendous lift in the back ribs, which further increases the circulation to the upper chest and breasts. It also allows the throat to relax and reduces elevated blood pressure.

Come into Salamba Sarvangasana II, with your sacrum firmly supported on the chair seat. Raise your legs up into a vertical position (9.4f). Lift your back ribs, move them toward your breastbone, and expand your chest. Bring your feet together. Extend your legs through your inner heels and the balls of your feet.

BADDHA KONASANA IN SALAMBA SARVANGASANA II. If you feel any strain in the lower back in Viparita Karani in Salamba Sarvangasana II, this variation releases that pressure and relaxes the abdomen. Bend your knees out to the sides and bring the soles of your feet together. Rest the outer edges of your feet on the chair back (9.4g).

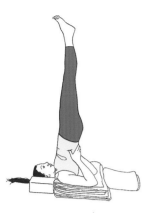

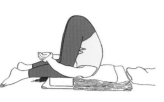

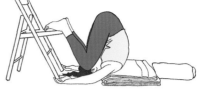

9.5A SALAMBA SARVANGASANA I   9.5B FINAL POSE   9.5C WITH CHAIR

9.5
Karnapidasana
Ear Pressure Pose

BENEFITS. This posture relieves low backache that may be experienced in Salamaba Sarvangasana I. It helps to draw the senses in from external distractions. It also benefits those with constipation.

PRACTICE. Set up as for Salamba Sarvangasana I, including folding your mat into fours and the blankets to the width of the mat. Place the two blocks, lengthwise and on their flat side, on either side of where your head will be. Assume Salamba Sarvangasana I (9.5a). Bend your knees and place them by the side of your head, one on each block. Wrap your arms around your legs (9.5b). Settle into the posture, allowing your upper back to round and your body to relax. Surrender quietly into the pose. When your back feels refreshed, return to Salamba Sarvangasana I.

CAUTIONS. If you are new to this pose or are unsure of whether your neck can support the weight of your body, start by keeping your hands on your back

KARNAPIDASANA WITH CHAIR. If you are working with Halasana with Chair (9.6d), hook your toes over the front edge of the chair. This does not take you so deeply into the pose, but it provides a quick and effective method of relieving a lower backache (9.5c).

9.6
Halasana
Plow Pose

BENEFITS. The dynamic lift of the trunk and spine and the corresponding expansion of the chest is part of what makes Halasana so powerful. It restores health to the pelvic organs, and can relieve the symptoms of cystitis, and realigns a displaced uterus. It relieves fatigue, calms the nerves, and regulates blood pressure. It also balances the endocrine system and keeps menstrual problems at bay. In addition it stimulates circulation to the facial muscles and skin and reduces the aging effects of wrinkles, tension, and dehydration.

PRACTICE. Continue from Salamba Sarvangasana I. Keeping your legs straight and your spine erect,

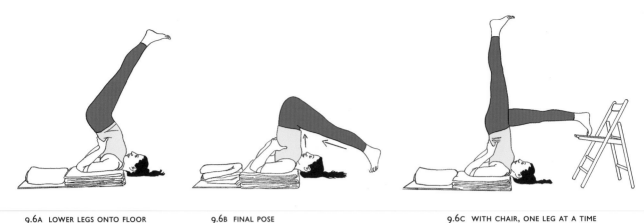

9.6A LOWER LEGS ONTO FLOOR   9.6B FINAL POSE   9.6C WITH CHAIR, ONE LEG AT A TIME

lower your legs over your head and onto the floor (9.6a). Walk your feet toward your head and tilt your pelvis back. If possible, your spine should be perpendicular to the floor. Bring your hands farther down your back toward your shoulder blades and press your thoracic spine in. This will bring your breastbone toward your chin (9.6b). Pull up through your inner groins so your side waist lengthens. Keep your thighs active by pulling your kneecaps up.

To come out: if you are using a strap, release it. Walk your feet toward your head. Supporting your back with your hands, bend your knees, and roll slowly back along your spine, vertebra by vertebra, onto the floor. Turn onto your right side and rest for a few breaths. Place your left hand on the floor and, without lifting your head, push up from your left hand and sit up.

CAUTIONS. Avoid all variations and modifications of Halasana during menstruation and if you have a neck injury or shoulder problem. If you are suf-fering from any kind of headache, wait until it has abated before practicing this posture. If you experience any neck discomfort or pain, there may be too much weight bearing down on your neck; bring your hands farther down your back and actively lift your spine higher. You can also work with your feet on a chair. If this does not alleviate your discomfort or pain, come down and add one more blanket to your stack.

HALASANA WITH CHAIR. Beginners: lower your legs, one at a time, onto the chair seat (9.6c, 9.6d). To come out, walk your feet toward the edge of the chair and come down as described for Halasana.

SUPTA KONASANA. In addition to the benefits of Halasana, this pose keeps the vaginal area healthy and treats hemorrhoids. It aids recovery following menstruation because it increases circulation to the uterus. Supta Konasana also strengthens the back muscles, helps correct a prolapsed or dis-

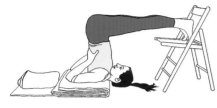

9.6D WITH CHAIR, FINAL POSE

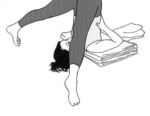

9.6E SUPTA KONASANA WITH BLOCKS

placed uterus, and lengthens and releases the hamstring muscles. However, do not practice it during the menstrual period.

Begin in Halasana. If you need support in Halasana, you may need an extra mat, as well as two blocks (9.6e) or two extra chairs (9.f). Set up your props so you can comfortably rest the tips of your toes on the props without rounding your back.

Spread your legs wide apart, keeping the soles of your feet upright (9.6g). Keep your spine erect and actively lift your back ribs with your hands. Draw the tops of your thighs away from your head, stretch and open the backs of your legs, and extend through your heels and up through your sitting bones. The center of the backs of your legs should face the ceiling. To come out, walk your feet back to center.

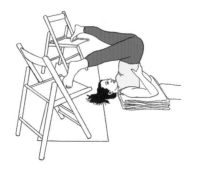

9.6F SUPTA KONASANA WITH CHAIRS   9.6G SUPTA KONASANA, FINAL POSE

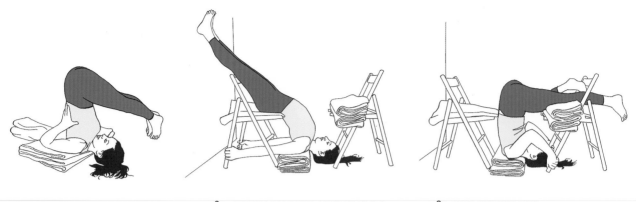

9.7A FINAL POSE   9.8A STARTING IN SALAMBA SARVANGASANA II   9.8B CLIMB THROUGH CHAIR

9.7
Parsva Halasana
Lateral Plow Pose

BENEFITS. When practiced regularly, Salamba Sirsasana (9.2d), Salamba Sarvangasana I (9.3f), and Halasana (9.6b) help prevent constipation. Parsva Halasana is also an effective method of exercising the colon. This pose creates elasticity in the spine and improves circulation in the breasts.

PRACTICE. You are ready to practice Parsva Halasana when you can do Supta Konasana from the floor, with the torso lifted and legs straight (9.6g). Begin in Halasana (9.6b). Press your left elbow down and walk your feet as far to the right as possible (9.7a). Keep your legs together. With your hands, raise your torso and stretch your legs. Keep your feet and ankles level with each other by drawing your right thigh back into its hip socket. Your knees and the center of your thighs should face the floor. Use your hands to help you press your back ribs in and to bring forward the right side of your torso. Revolve your chest and abdomen away from your legs. Feel how much space is created in the left breast when the torso is revolved to the right. Walk your feet back to

the center, and practice on the other side. To come out, walk you feet back to center and stretch your arms over your head. Roll out of the pose.

CAUTIONS. Do not practice this pose during the menstrual period.

9.8
Ardha Halasana
Half-Plow Pose

BENEFITS. Ardha Halasana recharges the adrenal glands, and allows the body, brain, and eyes to rest completely. It has the effect of lifting premenstrual fatigue and tension. When combined with forward bends, this pose can help to relieve a backache, and can help to stave off a migraine headache (practice with the eyes closed). Those with high blood pressure should practice Ardha Halasana for at least 5 minutes before going into Salamba Sarvangasana I (9.3f). This pose removes hardness and tension in the abdominal area. It is a very effective way to rest quickly.

PRACTICE. If you are coming into Ardha Halasana from Salamba Sarvangasana II, place a second chair across from and facing the other chair (9.8a).

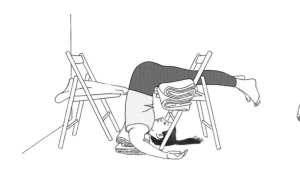

9.8c FINAL POSE FROM SALAMBA SARVANGASANA II

9.8d FINAL POSE

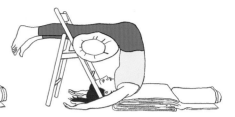

9.8e WITH THIGHS RAISED ON BOLSTER

If you have a long torso, place folded blankets across the chair seat to add height. Bend your knees over your head and climb your legs through the chair (9.8b). Rest your thighs on the support (9.8c).

At those times when Ardha Halasana is not preceded by Salamba Sarvangasana I or Salamba Sarvangasana II, lie with your shoulders on three blankets, your hips on a thickly folded blanket, and your head under the chair seat. Bend your knees up and over the seat. Maneuver your legs one at a time through the chair. Pull the chair toward you so the chair legs touch the blanket and the chair seat is directly over your head. Walk your legs away from you so your thighs are well supported (9.8d). With practice, this maneuver becomes effortless. However in the beginning, if you slide off the blankets, come down and start again with the shoulders a little farther in from the edge of the blankets.

If, despite the blankets, there is pressure on your neck, add another blanket, draw your breastbone slightly away from your head, or slide your legs an inch or two out of the chair. You may want to combine one or more of these three options.

Rest your arms on the floor outside the chair and relax them completely. Allow your whole body to release into the pose. Soften the muscles around your eyes and mouth. Allow the back

muscles to relax. Draw the crown of your head away from your neck and relax your throat. Allow your breath to be soft and quiet. Follow your exhalation and pause momentarily at the end of it until it disappears over the horizon. Allow your inhalation to follow quietly and naturally.

If you came into the pose from Salamba Sarvangasana II, ease your legs out of the Ardha Halsana chair and place your feet on the back of the Salamba Sarvangasana II chair. Then slide down. If you did not come in from Salamba Sarvangasana II, then back your legs, one at a time, out the of chair and roll down.

CAUTIONS. Avoid Ardha Halasana and its modifications when you are menstruating or if you are suffering from neck or shoulder problems.

ARDHA HALASANA WITH ROLLED WASHCLOTH. If you are working to reduce a migraine or to slow down an overactive thyroid gland, place a rolled washcloth under your head at the occipital bone as for Setu Bandha Sarvangasana II (8.10b).

ARDHA HALASANA WITH THIGHS RAISED ON BOLSTER. If you have fibroids, you will benefit from having the thighs raised higher to avoid abdominal compression. Place a bolster across the chair

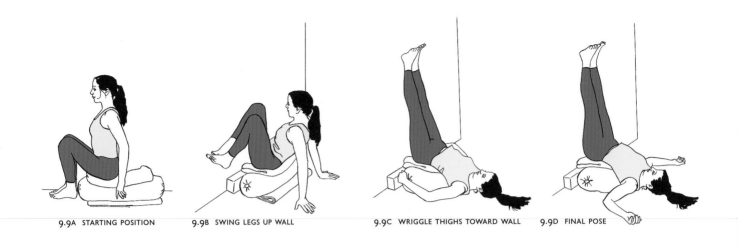

9.9A STARTING POSITION   9.9B SWING LEGS UP WALL   9.9C WRIGGLE THIGHS TOWARD WALL   9.9D FINAL POSE

seat. Rest the thighs on the bolster with the feet slightly apart (9.8e).

9.9
Viparita Karani
Inverted Relaxation Pose

BENEFITS. Viparita Karani is a surprisingly powerful pose. It aids the return of blood from the legs to the heart and the return of lymph fluid throughout the whole body. It relieves stress headaches, stabilizes blood pressure, and helps alleviate menstrual disorders. It also provides relief for the lower back and helps reduce soreness or inflammation in the abdominal area. But you don't have to have inflamed abdominal organs to enjoy this pose. Practice it at the end of a sequence or any time you feel like unwinding.

PRACTICE. Viparita Karani requires no effort to maintain, but skill and practice are required to get into the pose elegantly. Place two blocks horizontally, 3 feet apart, against the wall. Place a bolster, also horizontally, against the blocks. Place some folded blankets on top of the bolster so you

have sufficient height to support the back ribs and expand the chest. The longer your torso, the more blankets you will need.

Fold your mat into eighths and slip it half under the bolster, so the front edge is tilted up a little. This will stabilize the support and provide an extra lift for the chest.

Sit sideways on the blankets, with one hip touching the wall (9.9a). Place your hands onto the floor behind you. Pivoting on the pelvis, swing your legs up the wall (9.9b).

Curve your torso over the props. Rest the tops of your shoulders on the floor. Wriggle toward the wall to bring the backs of your thighs close to the wall (9.9c). Rest your arms out to your sides (9.9d). Relax.

To come out, bend your knees, press your feet against the wall, and slide backward into the room. Cross your legs and rest them on the support. Wait for a few moments. Turn over onto your side. Push with your hands to sit up, bringing your head up last. Coming out this way prevents an abrupt disturbance to the quietness that you have achieved.

CAUTION. Do not practice this pose during menstruation.

10

Back Bends: Opening the Heart

ONE OF THE REASONS for yoga's dramatic increase in popularity in recent years may be because it helps lift depression, an affliction that, in its many forms, has reached epidemic proportions in the United States. Our high-speed culture, with its worship of money, status, and celebrity, has led us away from our original nature. It also separates us from each other, so we become isolated, withdrawn, and anxious.

Yoga philosophy brings many helpful insights into how to connect with our true selves and heal our loneliness. One is the concept of dharma, a combination of destiny and duty. We each are born with an inherent aptitude to serve. Some are propelled to activism, others to business, still others to spirituality or creative endeavors. Honoring one's dharma leads to contentment and a sense of interconnectedness. Look into the face of someone who uses her unique talents to serve others, and you will see peace.

Yoga asana heals disturbances of the mind by changing the chemical balance within the brain and body. The mind, body, emotions, and spirit are so inextricably linked that when it comes to maintaining physical and mental health, compartmentalizing the different aspects of our being is not nearly as efficient as viewing ourselves as a whole. The physical counterparts of low self-esteem, habitual worry, and depression are slumped shoulders, a sunken chest, a tense jaw, and low energy. And this can work both ways: physical weakness or ill-health can also adversely influence our state of mind.

Yoga asana fall into broadly defined categories, and each category has an observably profound effect on the mind. Back bends lift the spirit. They open the chest and heart and direct the mind outward. As such, they make you feel positive and full inside. They also keep the spine supple and promote youthfulness, vitality, and energy.

Back bends also energize the reproductive system. They may even help to restore menstruation when it has stopped due to the retention of, or inability to express, strong emotions. They release tension in the pelvic region; they increase blood flow and therefore the supply of oxygen and nutrients to the uterus, ovaries and fallopian tubes. This increased blood flow, which is effective on a cellular level, releases blocked energy, can activate dormant sexuality, and reduces the likelihood of cramps and other menstrual problems.

General Cautions for Practicing Back Bends

When practicing the back bends presented in this chapter, remember to follow these guidelines.

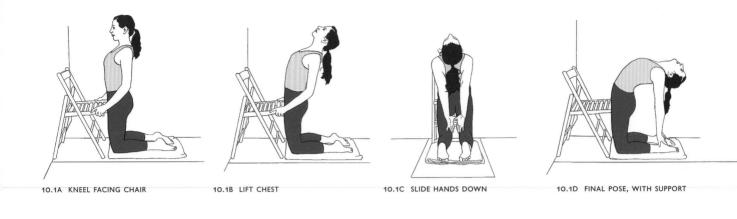

10.1A KNEEL FACING CHAIR   10.1B LIFT CHEST   10.1C SLIDE HANDS DOWN   10.1D FINAL POSE, WITH SUPPORT

Cautions are also included with each pose.

- If you are new to back bends, begin with care. One of yoga's most valuable rewards is emotional stability. If you are a beginning student, however, you may feel overstimulated after practicing back bends. To balance their exhilarating effects, include them in an overall monthly practice that incorporates all the other poses.

- Do not practice back bends if you are bipolar (manic depressive) during manic episodes, because they will make you more manic. Practice standing poses instead.

- Although it is always important to pay attention to your monthly cycle in relation to your yoga practice, this awareness is crucial with back bends. Fluctuating hormone levels result in fluctuating levels of flexibility. Sometimes the body is supple, energy levels are high, and back bends come more easily. At other times, you may experience stiffness and it will take you longer to get going. Supta Virasana, Surya Namaskar, Bharadvajasana, and standing poses are heating poses and, as such, will help prepare you for a back bend practice.

- Do not practice the active back bends during or for three days following menstruation.

10.1

Ustrasana
Camel Pose

BENEFITS. This exhilarating pose mobilizes the shoulder and ankle joints and counteracts stiffness in the spine. It opens and energizes the chest and lifts the spirits. It tones the pelvic organs, so when menstruation comes around the flow is neither excessive nor scanty and menstrual cramps are reduced.

PRACTICE. Place a chair with its back to the wall. Fold your mat into four and fold one blanket to mat width. Place the mat, with the blanket on top, on the floor in front of the chair. Kneel on the blanket, facing the chair, with your thighs touching the seat (10.1a). Separate your knees and feet to the width of your hips and point your feet straight back. Grip the sides of the chair seat and lift your entire torso up. Tuck your tailbone in. Roll your shoulders back and bring the points of your shoulder blades deep into your upper back. From within, vertically lift your breastbone and open your chest (10.1b).

Curve your spine in, and begin to arch back. Slide the backs of your hands down and press

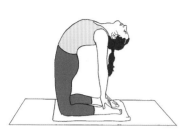

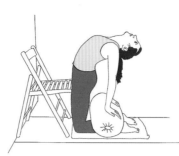

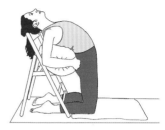

10.1E FINAL POSE, CLASSIC   10.1F WITH BOLSTER   10.1G WITH UPPER BACK SUPPORT

them against your inner thighs (10.1c). Move your hands from your inner thighs and, without sinking your chest, one by one stretch your arms down and reach for your heels. Point your fingers toward your toes (10.1d).

Press your thighs against the front of the chair. Spread your toes. Press your shins and the tops of your feet down. Turn your arms outward in their sockets. Coil your back ribs in toward your front ribs to further support and expand your chest. To prevent compressing the back of your neck, lengthen it and release the muscles around your upper back and shoulders down and away from your neck.

Continue to use your tailbone to press your pubic bone or the tops of your thighs against the chair. Take care not to squeeze your buttocks toward each other. Instead move the buttock muscles downward. This last action is the key to avoiding abdominal tension by maintaining a soft belly and a long lower back when practicing back bends. The more grounded you are at the base of the back bend (in this case, the shins and the tops of the feet), the greater will be your capacity for dynamically lifting and broadening the chest. Practice the classic pose without the chair when you have understood the integrative action of the spine and tailbone (10.1e).

To come out, press down through the thighs.

Using the firm support of your shoulder blades and maintaining the buoyancy of the chest, release your hands from your heels, place them on your hips, and swing your torso forward and up. Your head should come up last.

CAUTIONS. Do not practice Ustrasana if you are a beginning student or if you have a herniated disk, a migraine or tension headache, constipation, diarrhea, or hypertension.

USTRASANA WITH BOLSTER. If you find it difficult to reach the soles of your feet, place a bolster across your lower legs and drop your hands onto the bolster (10.1f)).

USTRASANA WITH UPPER BACK SUPPORT. Practice this modification if you are weak, if you have a tight upper back and shoulders, or you suffer from lower back pain. Place a bolster across the chair seat. Kneel with your back to the chair and your legs underneath it. Lean your elbows back onto the bolster, and curve your torso and head back. Arch over the bolster. Rest your head against the back of the chair (10.1g). Press your shins to the floor and push your thighs forward. Roll your shoulders back and press your shoulder blades into your back. Lift and open your chest.

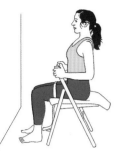

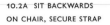

10.2A SIT BACKWARDS
ON CHAIR, SECURE STRAP

10.2B SLIDE THROUGH CHAIR

10.2C STRETCH LEGS, PRESS HANDS

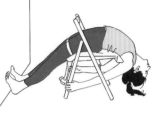

10.2D ARMS THROUGH CHAIR

10.2

Viparita Dandasana II
Inverted Staff Pose

BENEFITS. In this version of Viparita Dandasana, the chair provides the support needed to open the chest and mobilize the spine and shoulders without placing undue stress on the body. The pose is soothing to the lungs, heart, and brain cells. It helps those suffering from depression by promoting a feeling of well-being. In addition it opens ligaments behind the breasts, tones breast tissue, and prepares the spine for Urdhva Dhanurasana (10.4f) and other advanced back bends. It also stimulates the adrenal, thyroid, pituitary, and pineal glands and can help correct a prolapsed uterus. Regular practice of the pose reduces the likelihood of menstrual cramps.

PRACTICE. Place the chair facing into the room and about 2 feet from the wall. Place a nonslip mat on the chair seat. Sit on the chair seat, with your legs through the back. Secure a strap around the middle of your thighs to help prevent abdominal strain (10.2a). Slide through the chair until your tailbone is on the back edge of the seat (10.2b).

Hold the sides of the chair, lean back, and press your elbows into the chair seat. Curve back over the chair seat and allow your shoulder blades to just clear the front edge. Stretch your legs and place the soles of your feet on the floor against the wall.

Press the heels of your hands against the sides of the chair back and, against that resistance, bend your upper back farther around the front edge of the chair (10.2c). Slide a little further off the edge of the chair. Thread your arms through the front legs of the chair and hold the back legs (10.2d). Draw your breastbone toward your head. Feel your breast area stretching and opening. Beginning students stop here. Release your hands from the sides of the chair. Raise your arms, one at a time, over your head. Fold your arms and clasp your elbows (10.2e).

To avoid the weight of your arms dragging you toward your head, intensify the extension of your legs: extend your inner heels and the inner balls of your feet into the wall. Firm your kneecaps into your legs and draw them up into the thighs. Rotate your thighs in and press your shins toward the floor.

To come out, bend your knees. Grasp the chair back and slide your buttocks back into the center of the chair seat. Support your head with one hand (10.f). Press your other elbow into the chair and swing up, leading with your breastbone. Slide

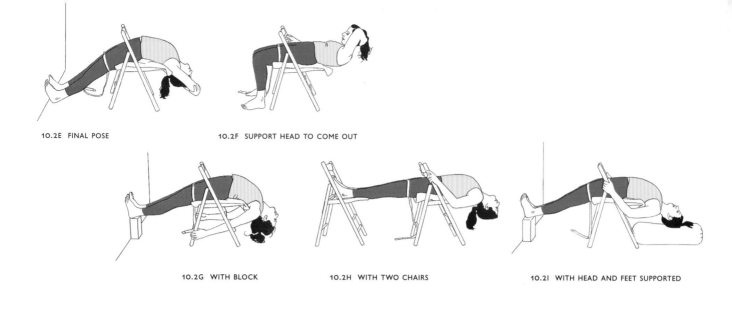

10.2E FINAL POSE   10.2F SUPPORT HEAD TO COME OUT

10.2G WITH BLOCK   10.2H WITH TWO CHAIRS   10.2I WITH HEAD AND FEET SUPPORTED

the chair toward the wall, and stretch your arms up the wall to release and lengthen your lower back.

CAUTIONS. Do not practice this pose if you have a herniated disk, a migraine or tension headache, diarrhea or constipation, or if you are menstruating. During menstruation, practice Viparita Dandasana II with head and feet supported.

VIPARITA DANDASANA II WITH BLOCK. If your lower back hurts, place a blanket under your waist and your feet on a block (10.2g). If you still have lower back pain, try Viparita Dandasana with Two Chairs (10.2h).

VIPARITA DANDASANA II WITH TWO CHAIRS. This variation mobilizes the upper back and shoulders and opens the chest. This posture is an effective alternative for beginners or those who are not able to practice this with one chair, due to rigidity of the dorsal spine and resulting lower back pain.

Position two chairs, facing in the same direction, with the front of one chair seat touching the back of the other. Place a folded nonslip mat on the front chair so it drops slightly over the front edge.

Climb through the front chair, with your feet on the floor between the two chairs. Place a strap around the middle of your thighs. Place your legs on the second chair, and slide through the one you are sitting on until your tailbone is resting at the back edge of the seat. Hold the sides of the chair, lean back, and press your elbows into the chair seat.

Allow your shoulder blades to just clear the front seat edge. Fully stretch your legs and flex your toes. Press the heels of your hands into the sides of the chair and, against that resistance, curve back around the edge of the chair (10.2h).

To come out, bend your legs, place your feet on the floor and swing up (leading with the breastbone) to sitting.

VIPARITA DANDASANA II WITH HEAD AND FEET SUPPORTED. Practice this version of Viparita Dandasana as an alternative to Salamba Sirsasana (9.2d) during menstruation. This is one of the poses that can help prevent insomnia during menstruation. In addition it soothes the heart and brain and allows for relaxation and deep, free breathing. Those with neck pain also benefit by having the head supported.

Support your head on a bolster and your feet on blocks, so that the feet are only a little lower than the hips. Secure a strap around the middle of the thighs. Curve back and stretch your legs away from you (10.2i).

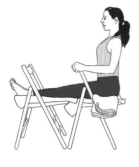

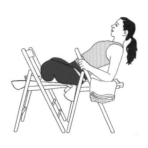

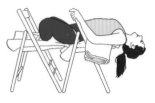

10.3A SIT IN DANDASANA
ON TWO CHAIRS

10.3B LEGS IN BADDHA KONASANA, LEAN
BACK ON ELBOWS

10.3C HOLD SIDES OF CHAIR,
ARCH BACK

10.3

Supta Baddha Konasana in Viparita Dandasana II
Bound-Angle Pose in Inverted Staff Pose

BENEFITS. This pose combines elements of an inversion (where the head is lower than the rest of the body), a back bend, and a strong pelvic stretch. It is wonderful to practice at any time, because it boosts energy and the immune system. The pelvic organs are provided with a fresh supply of blood. The ovaries, the adrenals, and the other endocrine glands are stimulated, and the body is better able to deal with stress and disease. This pose is useful if the monthly menstrual flow is scanty or sporadic or irregular, because flow blockages can be released by the increased circulation and the release of tension in the area. If menstruation has ceased altogether (a condition known as amenorrhea) and you are not pregnant or in menopause, the pose will help promote a healthy and regular menstrual flow.

PRACTICE. Position two backless metal folding chairs, facing in the same direction, with the front of one chair seat touching the back of the other.

To keep the chairs from sliding, place them on a mat. Put a folded mat on each chair seat. Fold a blanket lengthwise and place it across the seat of the front chair. Climb through the front chair and sit in Dandasana across both chairs (10.3a). Make sure that the two chairs remain touching throughout the pose.

Slide your pelvis through to the second chair and sit securely across both seats. Bend your legs out to the sides and bring the soles of your feet together. Secure them with a strap, as in Baddha Konasana (6.2a).

Position yourself so that, when you arch back over the chair, your shoulder blades are hooked over the front edge of the seat, and your sacrum is supported across the back of the first chair seat and the front of the second (10.3b).

Hold the sides of the chair and arch back (10.3c). Press your upper arms into the chair seat and lift your thoracic spine off the chair. Firm your shoulder blades into your upper torso. Draw your breastbone toward your head, and curve your torso back around chair seat. Place your arms underneath the overlapping blanket, and hang your elbows off the sides of the chair. Allow your inner thighs to open away from each other (10.3d).

When you have become proficient in this pose, that is, when you experience no back pain or discomfort either in the pose or as a result of it, then

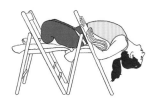

10.3D ARMS UNDER BLANKETS,
ELBOWS HANG OFF CHAIR

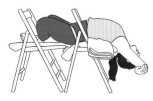

10.3E FINAL POSE

you can intensify the stretch through the abdomen and adrenal glands, as well as increase the arch of the upper spine and the opening at the shoulder joints, by folding your arms over your head (10.3e).

To come out, press your elbows into the chair seat. Initiating the action from your back ribs, swing up. Release the strap.

CAUTIONS. Do not practice this pose if you are a beginner, if you have a herniated disk, migraine or tension headaches, diarrhea, or constipation, or if it makes you feel dizzy.

10.4
Urdhva Dhanurasana
Upward-Facing Bow Pose

BENEFITS. Urdhva Dhanurasana quickly increases the heart rate and thereby improves circulation throughout the body. It strengthens the muscles of the abdomen and thighs, tones the abdominal organs, and stimulates the nervous system. In addition, it awakens the spine and increases its strength and flexibility. It generates feelings of elation and promotes courage and self-confidence.

Throughout the course of my yoga teaching career, I have come across many young women whose repressed anger has resulted in arrested menstruation (stress-related amenorrhea). If your period is delayed due to emotional factors or congestion, or if your periods have stopped altogether, back bends can help to bring your periods back on track by stimulating glandular activity. This pose also reduces the incidence of menstrual cramps.

PRACTICE. Lie on your back on your mat. Bend your knees and draw your feet close to your buttocks. Place your feet hip-width apart with the

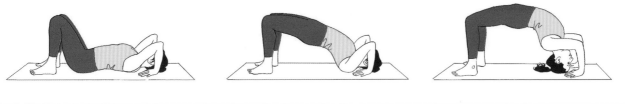

outer edges parallel. Bend your elbows and place your hands either side of your neck, with your fingers pointing toward your feet. Roll your elbows in, aligning them over your shoulders (10.4a).

Hold the floor well with your hands and feet. To do so, spread your fingers and open your palms. Then activate the arches of your feet. Press your heels and the balls of your feet down and lift your toes up. Exhale and raise your hips as high as possible (10.4b).

With another exhalation, raise your chest off the floor and come onto the crown of your head (10.4c). Keeping your elbows tucked in toward each other, roll your shoulders away from your ears. Retain the length of your torso from both ends: Lift your tailbone and, at the same time, extend it away from your lower back. Coil your shoulder blades into your upper back, bring your back ribs to vertical, and open your chest.

Before pushing up, allow your elbows to widen a little. Exhale, and push up into the pose, straightening your arms (10.4d). Use the shoulder blades, the back ribs, and the backs of your thighs to take you up, rather than initiating the action from the abdominal muscles. Learn to push up with equal vigor through the legs and arms. Pushing too hard with the arms may cause you to push into the throat, which can overstimulate the thyroid gland.

As women, we tend to fall into two camps: either our abdominal muscles are very hard and tight or they are slack and soft. Wherever you fall on the continuum, work carefully at the base of the pose. Keep your hands and feet well grounded: press down with your knuckles (at the base of your fingers), the balls of your feet, and your heels. Walk your feet in toward your hands (10.4e). Fully stretch your arms. Create a strong support for the pelvic organs by holding the pose firmly from the back ribs and sacrum. Press your back ribs in and move your chest away from your pelvis. Lift your tailbone and move the backs of your thighs up and toward your buttocks (10.4f) Remember that your arms and legs create the action and the spine receives the action. The lower spine should remain long and the abdomen and throat without strain. Feel the torso and hips opening and releasing from inside. Move in and out of this pose several times, until you are strong enough to hold it for 5 to 10 seconds.

Come out the same way that you went up—with awareness. If during the pose you walked your feet in, walk them back out before coming down. Return the crown of your head to the floor, with your chest lifted and your elbows in. Then

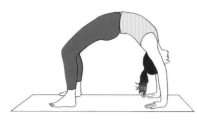

10.4D PUSH UP

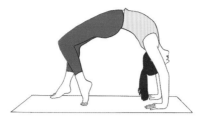

10.4E WALK FEET IN

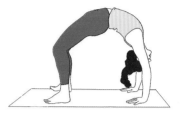

10.4F FINAL POSE

place the back of your head on the floor. Then slowly lower your trunk and pelvis to the floor. Release your arms and legs. Turn to the side. Push up with your hands.

CAUTIONS. Do not practice Urdhva Dhanurasana if you are a beginning student, if you are menstruating, or if you have a fever, high blood pressure, heart problems, chronic constipation, diarrhea, or any serious illness.

If your periods have stopped due to excess physical activity or low weight, do not practice this pose. Similarly do not practice it (even b-etween periods) if you are experiencing an exces-sively heavy or prolonged menstrual flow or short period cycles, until things return to normal.

URDHVA DHANURASANA WITH A BOLSTER AND BLOCKS. Urdhva Dhanurasana is a challenging pose. It requires developed upper body strength and sheer pushing power to get into it. If pushing up remains impossible, support your head and torso on a vertical bolster and your hands on two blocks propped against the wall at an angle of 45 degrees and on either side of the bolster (10.4g). At this stage, there is no need to go through the position on the crown of the head. Just push up (10.4h).

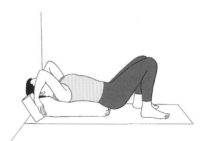

10.4G WITH BOLSTER AND BLOCKS, PLACEMENT

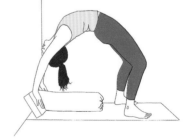

10.4H WITH BOLSTER AND BLOCKS, FINAL POSE

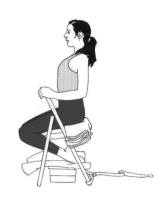

10.5

Kapotasana
Supported Pigeon Pose

BENEFITS. Kapotasana expands and opens the chest and tones breast tissue. It stretches the pelvic region and tones the abdominal organs, including the uterus, ovaries, and fallopian tubes. It helps keep the genital area healthy. This pose may help to bring on a period that has stopped or failed to start due to the retention of strong emotions.

PRACTICE. Place a backless metal folding chair on your mat. Stack three telephone books and slide them under the chair. Place a folded mat over the bar that runs between the back legs of the chair and over the telephone books; place another mat on the chair seat. Add a blanket that has been folded into a rectangle across the center of the chair seat. Secure a strap around the two front

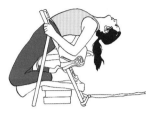

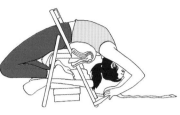

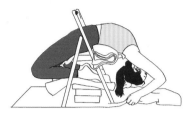

10.5B ARCH BACK   10.5C FINAL POSE: HOLDING BELT LOOP   10.5D FINAL POSE: HOLDING SIDES OF MAT

chair legs, leaving it slack. Extend the tail of the strap along the floor, in a straight line away from the chair.

Climb through the chair and bend your legs under it. Rest your lower shins on the bar and the tops of your feet on the telephone books (10.5a).

Draw your tailbone away from your lumbar spine. This action is important, because lengthening through the lumbar stops it from overbending or compressing. It also guards against pushing aggressively into the abdomen. Firm your back ribs and hook the points of your shoulder blades deep into your upper back. Roll your shoulders back and arch back over the edge of the chair (10.5b).

Keep your knees and feet close together. Stretch your arms over your head and take hold of the tail of the strap. Walk your hands along the tail until you reach the strap loop (10.5c). Keep your tailbone moving away from your lumbar spine and toward the backs of your thighs. Extend your thighs away from your pelvis and press your knees down, so your shins stay parallel to the floor. Curve your upper back farther around the edge of the seat.

If you have a toned body and are very flexible, you can try holding the two front chair legs. Alternatively you can hold the sides of a mat (10.5d). If you practice either of these alternative hand positions, keep your elbows shoulder-width apart. You can also press the heels of your hands into the sides of the chair.

To come out, bring your arms up and hold the sides of the chair. Press your elbows into the seat, hook your shoulder blades firmly into your back ribs, and swing your torso up, maintaining the back bend and the opening of the chest.

CAUTIONS. Do not practice Kapotasana if you are a beginning student or if you have back problems, high blood pressure, a fever, a migraine or tension headache, constipation, or diarrhea. Avoid this pose when menstruating, as well as throughout the month if your periods are very heavy or prolonged.

第21贴　正面　凯源-4色-WomandYoga-内页拼版.job

Pranayama: Exploring the Space Within

YOGIC BREATHING PRACTICES are called *pranayama*. The term is a composite of two Sanskrit words. *Prana* refers to the integrating energy that permeates all life. As such, it is both the breath itself and the life energy that allows the breath to be taken. *Ayama* means "extension." So *pranayama* means to extend, slow down, or control the breath. Ancient yogis taught that life expectancy could be determined by the length of one's breath and the rate of one's heartbeat. In addition they passed on to us important teachings about the vital interconnectedness of body, breath, and mind.

Accelerated heart rate, elevated blood pressure, and chronic anxiety are but a few of the problems we suffer from as a result of the pressures of the modern world. By controlling and steadying the breath, we control and steady the mind. We also reduce stress, stabilize the heart rate, and regularize blood pressure. In addition pranayama promotes a robust constitution; it keeps the lungs healthy and the body free from toxins. And for women, the practice can help the phases of the menstrual cycle go much smoother because pranayama regulates the endocrine system. Other functions in the body also become more efficient through the effect of increased carbon dioxide on the hormonal system. Metabolism, for instance, is regulated, as pranayama

improves the function of the pancreas. This can lead to weight loss for the overweight and stimulation of appetite for anorexics.

But most important, pranayama draws us inward, away from everyday events, and helps us reconnect with the divine, both within ourselves and beyond. It reminds us of who we really are—little points of radiant light, inextricably bound to each other by threads that form a sacred and shimmering web. Pranayama is like coming home.

General Cautions for Practicing Pranayama

When practicing the pranayama presented in this chapter, remember to follow these guidelines. Cautions are also included with each pose.

- It is important to establish good habits and avoid the mistakes that can easily be made with this deceptively powerful practice. Seek out good teachers for guidance with your pranayama.

- Do not embark on a pranayama practice until you have gained physical and emotional stability through asana.

- Pranayama can lift fatigue. However, if you are exhausted or are short of sleep or if you are upset, do not force yourself to practice. Instead practice a quiet sequence of reclining poses (such as those poses in chapter 8).

■ If you have a bad cold, skip pranayama until you feel better. If you simply have a congested nose (which is often caused by tension), part your lips and practice by inhaling through your mouth and exhaling as much as possible through the nose, until the nasal passages clear. Otherwise breathe through the nose throughout your practice.

■ Leave a space of at least 30 minutes between your pranayama and your asana practice.

■ Allow at least 3 hours to elapse between eating a heavy meal and doing pranayama.

■ Do not practice pranayama after a strong asana practice. Prepare for pranayama by practicing restorative poses (such as those in chapter 8).

■ It is important to relax the abdomen when practicing pranayama. If you are a beginning student, familiarize yourself with pranayama in a reclining pose, where it is easier to relax the abdomen and where it is easier to concentrate on the breath (sitting correctly requires strength and tremendous concentration). I also advise experienced practitioners to practice pranayama reclining when they are menstruating.

■ If you experience heat in the body or a sensation of pressure behind the eyes, either during or after pranayama practice, you may have used too much force. Call it a day and make sure you finish with a long, calming Savasana.

■ Saliva in the mouth signifies the formation of unspoken words or mental tension. Swallow at the end of the exhalation and take a few recovery breaths before proceeding.

Setting Up for Pranayama

First collect your props: one bolster, one nonslip mat, one or more blankets, and one bandage (or washcloth). Then set up in Savasana with Upper Back Supported (8.14g). Take your time. As soon as you begin folding the blankets, you have begun the process of realigning yourself with natural rhythms, whatever phase of the menstrual cycle you are in. Position yourself carefully and precisely. Allow yourself to settle into the pose. Completely relax your eyes, throat, and abdomen.

Wrapping the head keeps external distractions at bay. If you are a beginning student, you can place a folded head wrap or a small towel over the eyes, as described in chapter 8.

After Pranayama

When your pranayama practice is complete, turn to your side and, with a minimum of disturbance, sit up. If using a head wrap, slowly unwind the bandage from your head and drop it into your lap. Fold it to measure approximately 7 inches long. Lie down again and place a thinly folded blanket under your head and the folded head wrap over your eyes and rest for 5 to 10 minutes. If not using the head wrap, keep your eyes closed as you remove the support from under you and replace it with the folded blanket. When finished, turn to your right side, tuck your legs up underneath you, and stay quietly within yourself for a few minutes. Press your left hand down and sit up, bringing your head up last. Re-roll the bandage. Observe how you feel: mental activity should be almost nonexistent if your pranayama was practiced correctly.

ᎮᎮ.Ꭹ
Rhythmic Breathing

BENEFITS. You should first learn to breathe rhythmically and steadily before you take up the extended or interrupted breath.

Rhythmic Breathing helps prepare the upper body for pranayama practice. The lungs warm up, and the intercostals (the muscles between the ribs) become more pliable. A regular asana practice also releases tightness in the chest area. Rhythmic Breathing leads us smoothly into (and brings us carefully out of) each pranayama practice, so the nervous system does not get jolted or strained.

PRACTICE. Observe the gentle ebb and flow of your unconditioned breath. Notice that, as you let go of tension and holding patterns in the body, your breath becomes quiet and soft. Do not control it at this point but let the breathing breathe you.

When you are ready, deepen your breath a little: inhale slowly and easily and exhale slowly and easily. When you inhale, allow the chest to gently expand and the breastbone to lift without moving any other part of the body. Without using force, steer your exhalations toward an even, steady, leisurely flow. Observe and adjust the amount of air you take into your lungs so that they fill up and empty out evenly. Breathe rhythmically and gently.

CAUTIONS. Master Rhythmic Breathing before going on to the other breathing exercises.

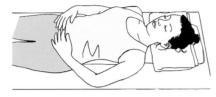

11.2A HANDS ON ABDOMEN

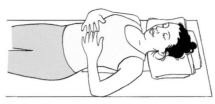

11.2B HANDS ON LOWER RIBS,
FINGERS TOUCHING

11.2C HANDS ON LOWER RIBS,
FINGERS MOVING AWAY

11.2

Breathing Awareness

BENEFITS. It is important to be aware of the difference between abdominal breathing and thoracic breathing before proceeding to other forms of pranayama in this book. When you are not practicing yoga, even when walking or running, the lungs neither fully inflate nor fully deflate. Breathing Awareness familiarizes you with how the chest feels and how the ribs move when you breathe deeply into the lungs. Breathing Awareness also trains you to breathe steadily without pumping the abdomen up and down, without tensing the diaphragm, and without agitating the brain or nervous system.

PRACTICE. Draw your senses inward and focus them on physical sensations.

Stage 1: Notice how the body responds to the breath: place your hands on your abdomen and take a couple of deep breaths (11.2a). Observe how it rises when you breathe in and sinks when you breathe out. Then consciously relax the belly, so the pumping action of the stomach becomes less extreme as you continue to breathe slowly and softly.

Now direct your breath to your chest: place your hands on your lower rib cage, middle fingers touching (11.2b). Relax the abdomen and watch how the lower ribs expand to the sides, moving the fingertips away from each other when you inhale and back toward each other when you exhale (11.2c).

Now place your hands at the top of the rib cage, with the middle fingers touching (11.2d). Deliberately deepen your inhalation, so the breath moves higher up into your chest. Notice how the in-breath not only moves the hands away from each other but also moves the hands up toward the throat, as the lungs fill with air and the chest expands (11.2e).

Watch the movement of the ribs as you exhale; just as they rise when you inhale, they fall when you exhale. Now exhale in such a way that the rib cage does not sink but remains firm and lifted as the air is expelled from the lungs. Keep the abdomen relaxed throughout.

Stage 2: Shift your focus to the back ribs. With your arms resting on the floor by your sides (and your upper arms turned out), bring your awareness to the back and sides of your torso as you breathe steadily and softly. Inhale and feel the sensation of the back ribs expanding into the bolster. Observe also how the side ribs expand out to the sides on the inhalation and return back to

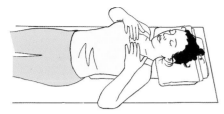

11.2D HANDS ON TOP RIBS, FINGERS TOUCHING

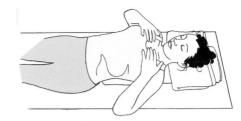

11.2E HANDS ON TOP RIBS, FINGERS MOVING AWAY

normal when the exhalation is complete. Allow the breath to touch (and observe the sensation of) the entire inner circumference of the rib cage.

Do not allow your shoulders to move up during this process. You can readjust them after your exhalation if they have crept up toward the neck. Roll your shoulders away from your neck; draw your breastbone and the sides of your upper chest to lift toward your head. Then inhale a little, exhale and empty the lungs, and start again with your inhalation.

When you have become familiar with the way the extended breath moves the rib cage from within, without creating tension in the face, throat, or stomach, you are ready for Ujjayi I and II.

CAUTION. Do not practice with force. When the breathing is too hard, pressure is placed on the brain, nerves, and lungs. If Breathing Awareness makes you tearful, you are not ready for pranayama. Focus on your asana practice and come back to it at a later date.

Feel free to return to Breathing Awareness as a separate practice any time you need a tactile reminder of thoracic breathing. For instance, if you have not practiced pranayama for a while, a session of Breathing Awareness can help get you going again.

11.3
Ujjayi I
Normal Inhalation, Extended Exhalation

BENEFITS. In general, the Ujjayi pranayamas generate vital energy, soothe the nerves, steady the mind, and remedy shortness of breath. When you focus on the sound of the breath, you become less distracted and less agitated.

The prolonged exhalation cleanses you emotionally and dissolves negativity. Extended exhalations relieve migraine headaches, lift fatigue, and reduce high blood pressure. During menstruation, exhalation—the breath of surrender—allows you to go with the flow. If you are cramping, use each exhalation to release pain and tension. Ujjayi I works well at the dentist too! Even though your mouth is open, focusing on the extended exhalation will help you relax and allow the dentist to get on with the job.

PRACTICE. Without using force, gradually lengthen and slow your exhalations. As you exhale, assume the best for the world. Allow the inhalation to follow the exhalation naturally and easily.

Without amplifying it, monitor your exhalation

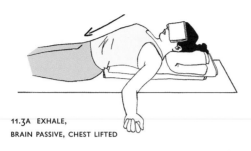

11.3A EXHALE,
BRAIN PASSIVE, CHEST LIFTED

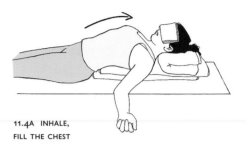

11.4A INHALE,
FILL THE CHEST

by listening to the sound that emanates from behind the breastbone: Trace it from its launch point (where your last inhalation ended) to its completion. The sound will tell you whether the breath is agitated or even, forced or easy. A break in the sound of the breath is a break in the flow of the breath. Let it take a few cycles to arrive at a rhythm that works for you.

As you focus on the exhalation, keep the brain passive and the chest lifted and open (11.3a). Keep your abdomen soft and your eyelids quiet throughout.

As your capacity to exhale increases, you may find that your inhalations also deepen. Allow this to happen naturally, still focusing primarily on the long, slow, soft exhalations. Allow each out breath to wash away your tensions, wherever they may be—in the fingers, in the feet, in the diaphragm, in the abdomen, or in the face.

CAUTION. If you experience any strain in the throat, tongue, eyes, or abdomen, or if your breath becomes mechanical, take some recovery breaths at the end of the exhalation and reestablish the calm of Savasana. When ready to resume, empty the lungs, inhale, and slowly, softly, and gently exhale.

If you are tearful or depressed at the end of this practice, wait a few weeks before attempting it again. Meanwhile continue with your asana practice.

11.4

Ujjayi II
Extended Inhalation, Normal Exhalation

BENEFITS. Ujjayi II, which emphasizes the inhalation, lifts the spirits and builds confidence. On an insecure day, practice long, slow inhalations and assume the best for yourself. Prolonging the inhalation increases oxygen to the body and boosts energy. It also helps those suffering from low blood pressure, asthma, and depression.

PRACTICE. Direct your awareness to the sensations of your inhalations and gradually allow them to get fuller and slower. Embrace your breath as it flows into your lungs: practice drawing the breath farther up toward the collarbones and spreading it to the outer corners of the chest. But prana cannot enter a closed space, so do not allow your chest to sink or compress. With the extended inhalation, allow the rib cage to expand and lift, opening from

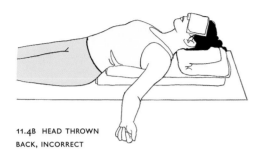

11.4B HEAD THROWN
BACK, INCORRECT

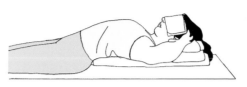

11.4C ADJUST THE HEAD

the center. Slowly fill up a bigger and bigger amount of space in your chest with air, until you reach your level of fullness for today (11.4a).

At the same time, relax the abdomen and maintain softness in the facial muscles. Allow the exhalation to follow, naturally and easily.

Without amplifying it, monitor your breath by listening to the sound that comes from behind the breastbone. The sound will tell you whether the breath is measured and even or jerky and tense. Breathe in such a way that the sound is smooth, continuous, and steady.

CAUTION. Do not allow the in-breath to suck in harshly through the nostrils. Sip the air in gently, so that it feels cool in the nostrils and sinus passages.

Do not allow the in-breath to lift the head back (11.4b, incorrect). This will have an agitating effect on the brain. If this occurs, at the end of your next exhalation adjust your head. Position your head carefully on the blanket, so it does not tip to the side and so your forehead slopes down slightly toward the chest (11.4c).

Ujjayi II can give you a headache if you try too hard. If you know that you are prone to hormonal migraines at predictable times of the month, stay away from extended inhalations at this time.

If you gasp for breath at the end of your exha-

lation, you attempted too deep an inhalation. Pause and take some normal breaths when you feel a strain or need to reestablish your relaxation. When you resume extended exhalation, take a little less during the next cycle and stay at that level for the duration of this practice.

11.5
Ujjayi III
Extended Inhalation, Extended Exhalation

BENEFITS. Ujjayi III pranayama brings about a combination of different effects. It strengthens your ability to focus and gives you energy. At the same time the mind becomes quieter and more peaceful, as the sounded breath settles into an even, steady rhythm. And when the mind starts following the sound of the breath, you may realize that all living things on the planet are breathing the same breath.

PRACTICE. Gradually allow both your inhalations and your exhalations to become slower and deeper. Take a full easy inhalation. Exhale smoothly and completely. Gradually prolong both the inhalations and the exhalations. As you

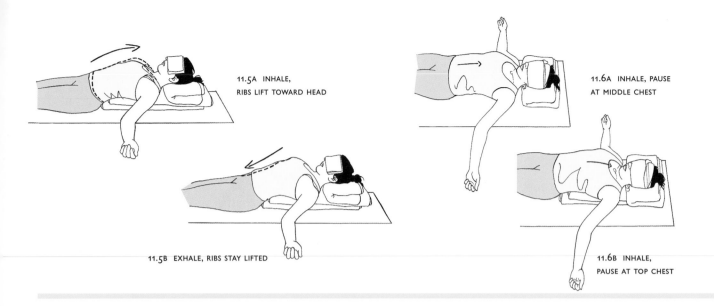

11.5A INHALE, RIBS LIFT TOWARD HEAD

11.5B EXHALE, RIBS STAY LIFTED

11.6A INHALE, PAUSE AT MIDDLE CHEST

11.6B INHALE, PAUSE AT TOP CHEST

inhale, allow the ribs to lift toward the head and to expand out from the center (11.5a). As you exhale, hold the diaphragm firmly up under your lower ribs and maintain the lift of the rib cage (11.5b). Observe the lungs carefully: breathe an even amount of air into each lung; exhale evenly from each lung.

Follow the sound of the breath: if your mind wanders, allow the sound to bring you back to yourself. Measure your breath by observing the sound: steer the breath so that the inhalations are the same length and velocity as the exhalations.

Breath delicately and gently. Not only is each breath precious, so too are the transitions between the incoming and the outgoing breath. Make sure that the exhalation is complete and that the inhalation follows smoothly and without effort. Similarly have the transition between the incoming breath and the outgoing breath be rhythmic and easy. Just as an incoming wave breaks against the shore and rolls back to join the sea, so the breath is a continuum of flowing movement.

CAUTIONS. If you become breathless, pause and take some recovery breaths at the end of your exhalation. If you experience tightness in the chest, pull back a little and don't attempt so deep

a breath next time. Find your own balance of focus and softness.

11.6

Viloma I
Interrupted Inhalation, Normal Exhalation

BENEFITS. Viloma pranayamas, in which the breath is interrupted, are a more refined pranayama than Ujjayi, although the extended breath can be easier to manage when you inhale and exhale in stages. When you practice interrupted flow, you become capable of longer breaths over time.

Viloma I nurtures and supports the nervous system and brings a sense of quiet well-being. It can be very helpful during menstruation or any time when energy is low. It is helpful for those with low blood pressure. Viloma I also reduces mood swings during the premenstrual phase and helps to correct an irregular menstrual flow.

PRACTICE. Exhale completely. Introduce your pauses on a gradient: inhale slowly and deeply and pause at the middle of your chest for a few seconds

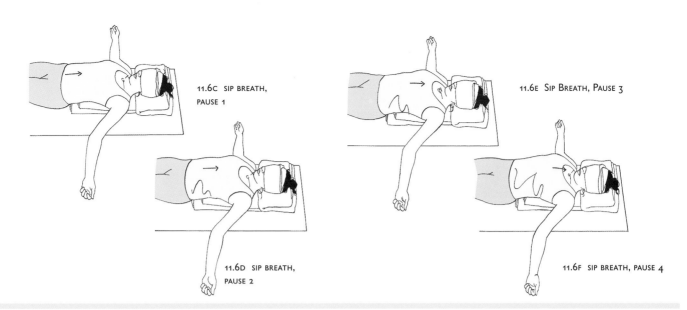

11.6C SIP BREATH, PAUSE 1

11.6E SIP BREATH, PAUSE 3

11.6D SIP BREATH, PAUSE 2

11.6F SIP BREATH, PAUSE 4

(11.6a) and again at the top of the chest for a few seconds (11.6b). Repeat this for a few cycles.

When you are ready, introduce more pauses, until you are sipping the breath in and pausing three or four times each cycle (116c through 11.6f). Inhale either to the breastbone or, if you can do so without strain, to the collarbones. The last retention could be longer than the previous ones.

Continue in this manner, inhaling and pausing, slowly filling the lungs (not the belly and not the head) without force. Watch for disturbances in the shoulders, eyes, temples, and throat. Make sure the tip of the tongue is not pressing the roof of the mouth or the back of the upper teeth. Let it rest lightly on the lower palate. Take some recovery breaths at the end of each cycle, and begin again with an exhalation.

CAUTION. Do not practice Viloma I if you have a migraine headache. Always stop before you reach your limit or if you feel fatigued.

11.7
Viloma II
Normal Inhalation, Interrupted Exhalation

BENEFITS. Viloma II calms and quiets the brain. It relaxes the body and can reduce high blood pressure. It helps reduce mood swings and irritability. Regular practice benefits those with a heavy or prolonged menstrual flow.

BEGINNING. Slip gently into Viloma II by introducing the pauses on a gradient. Exhale completely. Inhale deeply and then slowly exhale. Pause when the exhalation is complete. Then inhale again, slowly exhale half the volume of your breath, and then pause (11.7a). Exhale the second volume of breath, and pause again when the exhalation is complete (11.7b). Keep going this way, gradually introducing more pauses, until you are exhaling in three or four stages (11.7c through 11.f).

PRACTICE. Develop your awareness of this pranayama by close observation: make sure the chest is held firm (but not tight) when you exhale, and softly, softly does it! Be as gentle as you can with

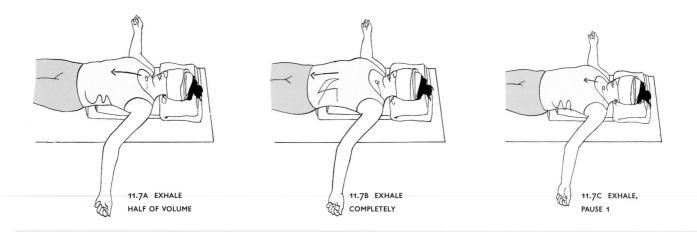

11.7A EXHALE
HALF OF VOLUME

11.7B EXHALE
COMPLETELY

11.7C EXHALE,
PAUSE 1

each exhalation. Think of the pause at the end of the exhalation as a moment of suspension in time. With each pause in the breath, center into the calm of your deeper self.

Don't make a big deal of the inhalation; that is, don't fill right up the collarbones with a heavily sounded breath. You need to inhale deeply, but you will be better able to handle the interrupted out-breath if the inhalation is a little easier.

When each cycle is complete, take some recovery breaths, where the exhalations are slightly longer than the inhalations.

Caution. Do not practice Viloma II beyond the point where you feel out of breath, tired, or mentally strained.

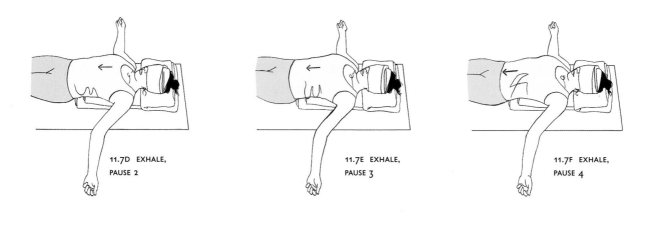

11.7D EXHALE,
PAUSE 2

11.7E EXHALE,
PAUSE 3

11.7F EXHALE,
PAUSE 4

12

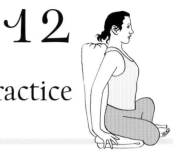

During Your Period: Effortless Practice

THE FOLLOWING three chapters describe practice sequences that you can use during the various phases of your monthly cycle. The sequence detailed in this chapter consists of poses to restore you during your bleeding phase. Chapter 13 gives a sequence for the days after your period, to help rebuild blood and energy. Chapter 14 gives a sequence of pranayama (breathing exercises) to practice throughout the month, to help you maintain vibrant good health and hormonal equilibrium at every stage of your cycle.

As we have already seen, the menstrual cycle is pretty much ignored in the Western world, despite its capacity for connecting us to the mystery of creation. No one made a fuss over me when my periods first started, and likewise no one took much notice of my mother's cycles. In fact, in our family and in most of the families I knew growing up, menstruation was not mentioned much at all. Perhaps if menarche, the first period, was celebrated in some way and the cyclic nature of women's physiology was respected, we would be more certain of our innate female power. What young girl would not enjoy a special treat—a show or concert or afternoon tea at the Ritz—to mark the occasion and to acknowledge her coming of age? On a purely practical level, when we pay attention to our hormonal rhythms and honor menstruation with appropriate actions on a regu-

lar basis, our cycles, our fertility, and our future pregnancies are strengthened and supported. Even menopause will go smoother if we take care of ourselves intelligently all the way along.

The spectrum of menstrual experience runs the gamut. Many women feel just fine. Others experience any number of symptoms, ranging from mild to extreme. Either way, women may find their overall health deteriorating if they are unable to rest and recuperate during menstruation.

Traditionally women chose rest and seclusion at this time. In ayurvedic custom, for instance, Indian women disturb themselves as little as possible during menses; they even refrain from bathing or washing their hair. This is probably unworkable for most of us, although it wouldn't be a bad idea to avoid excessively hot baths when bleeding is at its heaviest. In order to ensure that the body experiences the least degree of intrusion, consider taking a shower instead. Whenever possible, gather your energies and allow the menstrual process to take place undisturbed by external events. Ayurveda even advises against massage at this time, as it interferes with menstruation's natural balancing mechanism. Do not expose yourself to the cold. Spend some time alone, at least during the heaviest phase of your period. Reschedule business or social appointments to a later date. Give yourself a break from cooking and housework. Respect this time. In Native American tradition, a woman is considered to be at her most powerful psychically and spiritually when she is menstruating.

Watch the quality of your thoughts, dreams and visions. Reflect on time passing and on the times that are to come. But although rest is important, too much lying around can leave you feeling sluggish and dull. Tuning in to the ebb and flow of hormonal rhythms does not mean you should take to your bed; just slow down and nurture yourself a little for those few days. Yoga can provide you with the means of slowing down and—dare I say it—even enjoying the cleansing phase of the cycle. By establishing a calming yoga practice during menstruation, you realign yourself with the cycles of nature and maintain your health.

Practice

If you already have a regular and/or a vigorous yoga practice, I recommend that you stop doing it while you are bleeding, because strenuous exercise will deplete you rather than energize you at this time. If you are attending a yoga class, be sure to let your teacher know that you are having a period. Do not practice the inverted poses when menstruating, as it is damaging to do anything that prevents the menstrual blood from flowing. Likewise, standing poses, active back bends, and the strong twisting poses are best left until menstruation is over, as their practice disturbs *apana vayu,* the vital energy in the lower abdomen that supports elimination.

There are a few exceptions: Utthita Trikonasana, when practiced with the support of the wall to minimize exertion, can help reduce menstrual cramps (see chapter 19). Similarly Ardha Chandrasana, practiced with wall support, relieves menstrual cramps. Ardha Chandrasana with the leg supported is less strenuous still and can also reduce a heavy menstrual flow (see chapter 20). The standing forward bend poses—Uttanasana, Adho Mukha Svanasana, and Prasarita Padottanasana—can also be beneficial during menstruation. Practiced with the head supported, they relieve tension and calm the mind as well as help reduce cramping and low back pain. They appear in many of the sequences presented in this book.

Practice this restorative sequence during your period to ensure that you get the rest you need. The sitting poses in section I provide relief for women who feel achy or heavy in the legs and pelvis. In sections II and III, the combination of reclining poses and forward bends create a synergistic effect that fortifies the nervous system, restores depleted energy, and allows the mind to experience a quiet inner release. Follow the guidelines for setting up the seated forward bends given in chapter 7, but practice them during menstruation with a softer focus; sense the activity in the legs, rather than working to lengthen the hamstrings. Your primary intention should be to avoid stress or stimulation. Practice the reclining back bends (in section IV) to replace inversions.

Additionally, since you are not following your normal regimen now, you could take some time to work quietly on areas that you might ordinarily not have time to practice, such as the shoulders or hips. For instance, Gomukhasana and Paschima Namaskarasana are recommended by Geeta Iyengar as poses that can be safely practiced during menstruation. They are not strenuous and do not interfere with the menstrual flow. Add Urdhva Baddangullyasana in Virasana to these two poses and, with the addition of Setu Bandha Sarvangasana II, you have an additional sequence. You can also practice them at the beginning of the menstrual sequence that follows.

Practice time: 60–90 minutes

I: For Repose

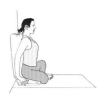

6.2e
Baddha Konasana
Against Wall
1–5 minutes

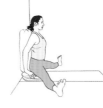

6.3c
Upavistha Konasana
with Wall and Bolster
1–2 minutes

II: For Relaxation of the Nerves and the Uterus

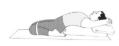

8.4h
Supta Virasana
with Arms Above Head
1–2 minutes, increasing
to 5 minutes or more with
practice

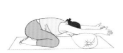

6.9e
Adho Mukha Virasana
with Bolster
30–60 seconds

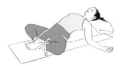

8.2c
Supta Baddha Konasana I
5–10 minutes

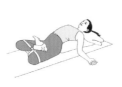

8.5f
Matsyasana with Bolster
(continuing practice)
30–60 seconds or more,
change legs,
30–60 seconds or more
or

8.6a
Supta Swastikasana
(beginning practice)
2 minutes, change legs,
2 minutes

III: To Calm the Brain and Soothe the Abdomen

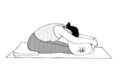

7.4e
Paschimottanasana with
Horizontal Bolster
20–30 seconds

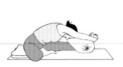

7.1k
Janu Sirsasana with
Horizontal Bolster
30–60 seconds, each side

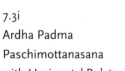

7.2f
Triang Mukaikapada
Paschimottanasana with
Horizontal Bolster
(continuing practice)
30–60 seconds, each side.
If you find this difficult,
repeat Janu Sirsasana with
Horizontal Bolster (7.1k).

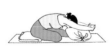

7.3i
Ardha Padma
Paschimottanasana
with Horizontal Bolster
or Chair (continuing practice)
30–60 seconds, each side
or

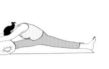
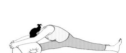

6.12a
Adho Mukha
Swastikasana
(beginning practice)
30–60 seconds, change legs,
30–60 seconds

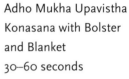

6.4d
Parsva Upavistha
Konasana with Bolster
20–30 seconds,
each side

6.5c
Adho Mukha Upavistha
Konasana with Bolster
and Blanket
30–60 seconds

7.4e
Paschimottanasana
with Horizontal Bolster
3–5 minutes

IV: For Hormone Balance and to Rest the Nerves

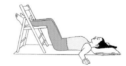

10.2i
Viparita Dandasana II with
Head and Feet Supported
5 minutes

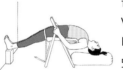

8.10a
Setu Bandha
Sarvangasana II
3–8 minutes

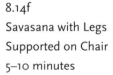

8.14f
Savasana with Legs
Supported on Chair
5–10 minutes

13

For the Days After Your Period: New Beginnings

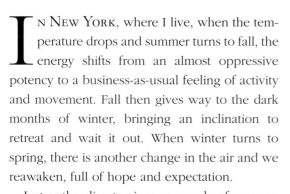

IN NEW YORK, where I live, when the temperature drops and summer turns to fall, the energy shifts from an almost oppressive potency to a business-as-usual feeling of activity and movement. Fall then gives way to the dark months of winter, bringing an inclination to retreat and wait it out. When winter turns to spring, there is another change in the air and we reawaken, full of hope and expectation.

Just as the climate gives us a cycle of seasons, so women have their own internal seasons, which take them through the menstrual cycle. And just as we all react differently to changes in the weather, the menstrual cycle affects each woman differently. For many women, menstruation is barely noticed. Others are miserable. Still others may recognize, however fleetingly, that the cycle of creation and dissolution that plays out every month in their cells reflects a larger rhythmic pulse.

The menstrual cycle divides into three phases. Phase I, the follicular, or the building up phase of the cycle, actually begins during the last few days of the previous, luteal phase. The follicles begin releasing estrogen, slowly at first, from about day three of the cycle (day one being the first day of bleeding). The days leading up to ovulation are a time of renewal and expectation. Just as in early spring the sap rises and buds appear on the trees, carrying the seeds of new growth,

so during this part of the menstrual cycle the egg develops in the ovary, and the lining of the uterus thickens in preparation for the fertilized egg.

Phase II, the ovulatory phase, is a process of two or three days of surging hormonal activity that results in ovulation. Ovulation itself occurs around day fourteen of the menstrual cycle, at the midpoint, corresponding to high summer. The matured egg bursts out of its follicle, and sensual and sexual desires are heightened. This is a time of fertility and enhanced mental and emotional receptivity to the world outside. Many women experience a sense of excitement and feel a surge of creativity around this time.

Phase III is the luteal, or letting out, phase of the cycle. An egg is released into the fallopian tubes and, if it is fertilized, it goes down to be implanted in the warmth and protection of the uterus. If fertilization does not take place, the endometrial lining begins to detach from the uterine wall. Just as the leaves on the trees are shed in order for new life to begin, the endometrial lining, along with the unfertilized egg and other secretions, are sloughed off. Menstruation, like winter, is a time to draw inward and gather energy.

Ayurveda recognizes the three days following menstruation as a transitional phase. It is worth paying attention to how you feel in the days following your period. After the cleansing and balancing that takes place during menstruation, many women feel renewed and look forward to new beginnings. Some may even experience an emotional response similar to the excitement following the birth of a baby. Others may feel a little tired, and still others, particularly if they have had an excessive or prolonged menstrual flow, feel washed out and exhausted. Where fatigue is combined with feelings of elation, a woman may tend to overdo things, and this may tax her inner reserves.

Practicing an appropriate sequence of yoga poses can help to balance the system and restore energy. Once a student of mine arrived for class complaining that her legs were hurting and she felt exhausted. It transpired that not only had her period just finished, but that morning she had been to the gym for a strong workout. Some restorative poses and supported inversions (the sequence follows) revived her. It was a learning experience for her. The next month she postponed the gym for a few days and practiced this sequence.

Use your yoga practice to honor this phase of the cycle and embrace the fresh start that menstruation has provided. Build up your energy gradually, and counterbalance the increased internal activity that occurs as the body makes the adjustment from winter to spring.

Practice

The following sequence helps the nervous system and the uterus recover from menstruation. Practice it for three days following menstruation (whether you feel tired or not), when there is no longer any residue of menstrual flow. Your practice at this time should be focused on the inversions.

The standing forward bend poses in section I, where the head is supported, calm the mind. They also prepare you for the inversions. In particular, in section II, Upavistha Konasana and Baddha Konasana in Salamba Sirsasana, and in section IV, Upavistha Konasana and Baddha Konasana in Salamba Sarvangasana I and Supta Konasana circulate blood around the reproductive organs and relax the uterus. Salamba Sirsasana, when you are able to practice it without strain, also stimulates the pituitary gland. (This has particular relevance for women with fertility issues, because the pituitary gland releases the hormones that trigger the development of follicles, which begin to develop on the ovaries from the first day of bleeding.)

Look at the suggested timings for these inverted poses, and make sure you don't run out of steam and have to come down before you get to the variations, because the variations are important. Salamba Sarvangasana I flushes the breasts with new blood and oxygen after the stasis and possible inflammation that takes place in the breasts during the premenstrual phase. This posture should be part of every woman's routine as a preventative measure against breast cancer, particularly during times of hormonal activity or growth spurts (puberty, pre- and postmenstruation, pregnancy and postnatal, and during breast feeding).

The supported back bend in section III, Viparita Dandasana, provides a welcome boost of energy at this time in a way that doesn't overexert the system.

Taken together, the postures in this sequence ensure a smooth transition from the active bleeding phase of the cycle to phase 1, the proliferative phase. They stabilize and support hormone activity and encourage the healthy functioning of the subsequent menstrual cycles.

Practice time: 60–90 minutes

I: To Reawaken the Body and Calm the Mind

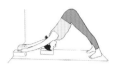

6.9c
Adho Mukha Virasana
30–60 seconds

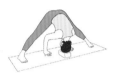

5.5g
Adho Mukha Svanasana
with Head Support
30–60 seconds

5.4h
Uttanasana with Head
Support
1 minute

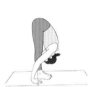

5.15f
Prasarita Paddottanasana
with Head on Block
1 minute

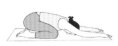

5.4c
Uttanasana
10 seconds

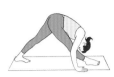

Step left foot back
to 5.12e
Parsvottanasana
20–30 seconds

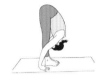

Step forward
to 5.4c
Uttanasana
10 seconds

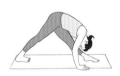

Step right foot back
to 5.12e
Parsvottanasana
20–30 seconds

Step forward
to 5.4c
Uttanasana
10–20 seconds

II: To Relax the Uterus and Support the Menstrual Rhythm

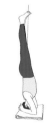

9.2d
Salamba Sirsasana
(continuing practice)
1–5 minutes
or
5.15f
Prasarita Paddottanasana
with Head on Block
(beginning practice)
1 minute

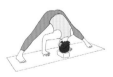

9.2g
Upavistha Konasana
in Salamba Sirsasana
15–20 seconds

9.2h
Baddha Konasana
in Salamba Sirsasana
15–20 seconds

6.9c
Adho Mukha Virasana
20–30 seconds

III: To Boost Energy

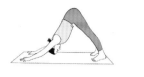 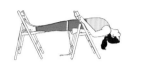

5.5d
Adho Mukha Svanasana
30–60 seconds

10.2h
Viparita Dandasana II
with Two Chairs
30–60 seconds, increasing
to 5 minutes with practice

6.17a
Supported Bharadvajasana II
20–30 seconds, each side

IV: For Recovery and Balance

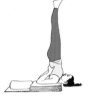

9.3f
Salamba Sarvangasana I
2–5 minutes, increasing
with practice

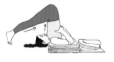

9.3j
Upavistha Konasana
in Salamba Sarvangasana I
15–20 seconds

9.3k
Baddha Konasana
in Salamba Sarvangasana I
15–20 seconds

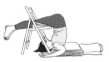

9.6b
Halasana
1–5 minutes

9.6g
Supta Konasana
30–60 seconds

9.8d
Ardha Halasana
5 minutes

V: To Calm the Nerves and Rest the Brain

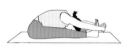

7.4c
Paschimottanasana
20–30 seconds

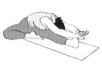

7.1f
Janu Sirsasana
30–60 seconds, each side

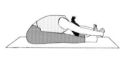

7.4c
Paschimottanasana
3–5 minutes

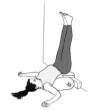

9.9d
Viparita Karani
5 minutes

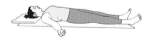

8.14d
Savasana
5–10 minutes

Breath Awareness: Focusing the Mind

AN ENHANCED OPPORTUNITY for self-awareness is one of the great gifts of the menstrual cycle. And when pranayama, yoga's breathing practices, are fine-tuned to the ups and downs of the month, a woman's understanding of herself can be further refined. Some women feel more introverted during menses, and the natural tendency to focus inward may be better appreciated when it is partnered with the breath.

Although all the pranayamas in this book can be practiced during menstruation—or indeed at any time throughout the month—you may find some more helpful than others as you become more sensitive to the fluctuations of your cycle. The breath can connect you with feelings held deep within muscle tissue. It can also release you from bondage and pain. The long, soft exhalations of Ujjayi I can relieve menstrual cramps, tense abdominal muscles, and constipation, especially if you let the tension remind you to exhale more deeply and slowly. The sense of relief that some women feel at the onset of menstruation can also be partnered with Ujjayi I.

During the premenstrual phase, when it is common for unresolved emotional problems to bubble to the surface, a session of focused deep breathing can help you balance and center.

Viloma II can be especially calming to the nervous system around this time.

Ujjayi II and Viloma I work well at any time to boost energy and dispel anxiety. Viloma I and Viloma II, practiced throughout the month, also benefit those with heavy, prolonged, or irregular periods.

Practice

The best time to practice is early in the morning, ideally before the rest of the world wakes up. Always prepare for each breathing exercise or pranayama practice by doing a few supported reclining poses, such as Supta Baddha Konasana I and Supta Virasana for a few minutes each to open the chest and release tension in the lungs. If you practice pranayama later in the day, start your practice with the restorative sequence in section I. It will help you to change gears and relax. Make sure you have your yoga kit at hand before beginning your practice, and take care that you do not get distracted as you move from pose to pose or rearrange your props. Direct your attention away from any preoccupations or worries, and let go of physical tension. As you progress through the restorative sequence, each pose should start at a deeper level of relaxation than the preceding one.

Once you have calmed yourself, you will be free to focus on the subtleties of the breath.

There are seven pranayama techniques presented in this book. Each one is a separate and complete practice. Experienced practitioners may combine several pranayamas in any given session.

Make sure you are comfortable and thoroughly familiar with Rhythmic Breathing and Breathing Awareness before proceeding with the other pranayama techniques. Rhythmic Breathing gives you the basics of conscious, steady, and easy breathing. Set up Savasana with Upper Back Supported for all pranayama practices in this book. Set aside 10 to 20 minutes for practice, including 5 to 10 minutes for Savasana at the end. Rhythmic Breathing leads you into and eases you out of each pranayama practice. Breathing Awareness introduces you to thoracic breathing and will help you understand how the ribs move and how the breath feels when you breathe into different parts of the torso and chest. Set up for Breathing Awareness in Savasana with Upper Back Supported. Set aside a practice time of 15 to 20 minutes, including

3 to 4 minutes of Rhythmic Breathing before and after Breathing Awareness, and 5 to 10 minutes of Savasana to finish.

Ujjayi I can also be practiced in Supta Swastikasana with Blankets or Supta Baddha Konasana II to relieve menstrual cramps or a heavy menstrual flow.

Just as your awareness of the poses is honed through repeated practice, so too will your concentration skills in pranayama develop over time. To enhance this process, wrap your head to shut out distractions. Beginners may, if they wish, cover the eyes with a folded head wrap or small folded towel. When you are familiar with this practice, you may also wrap the eyes. At the end of each pranayama practice, remove the head wrap, and finish your practice in Savasana, with the eyes lightly covered. For more information about wrapping the head, see chapter 8.

Practice whichever of the following sections, A through E, corresponds to your needs. See chapter 11 for recommendations on which pranayama to practice when.

I: PREPARING FOR PRANAYAMA WITH RESTORATIVE POSES
Practice time: 30 minutes

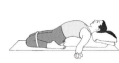

8.4c
Supta Virasana
30 seconds–5 minutes

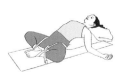

8.2c
Supta Baddha Konsana I
5–10 minutes

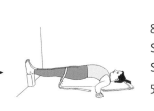

8.10a
Setu Bandha
Sarvangasana II
5–8 minutes

II: Practicing Pranayama

A: For Tension Relief
Practice time: 20–30 minutes

11.1
Rhythmic Breathing
3–4 minutes

→

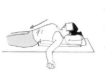

11.3a
Ujjayi I
10 or more cycles

→

11.1
Rhythmic Breathing
3–4 minutes

B: To Boost Energy and Lift the Spirits
Practice time: 20–30 minutes

11.1
Rhythmic Breathing
3–4 minutes

11.4a
Ujjayi II
10 or more cycles

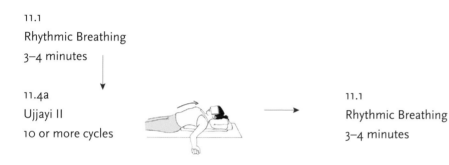

→

11.1
Rhythmic Breathing
3–4 minutes

C: To Strengthen the Nerves and Calm the Mind
Practice time: 20–30 minutes

11.1
Rhythmic Breathing
3–4 minutes

11.5a & 11.5b
Ujjayi III
10 or more cycles

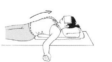 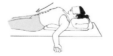

11.1
Rhythmic Breathing
3–4 minutes

D: To Dispel Anxiety and Promote Inner Calm

Practice time: 20–30 minutes

11.1
Rhythmic Breathing
3–4 minutes

11.4a
Ujjayi II
3–5 cycles

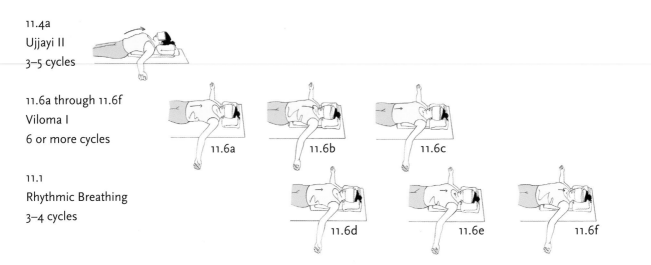

11.6a through 11.6f
Viloma I
6 or more cycles

11.1
Rhythmic Breathing
3–4 cycles

E: To Reduce Irritability and Soothe the Nerves

Practice time: 20–30 minutes

11.1
Rhythmic Breathing
3–4 minutes

11.3a
Ujjayi I
3–5 cycles

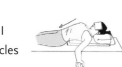

11.7a through 11.7f
Viloma II
6 or more cycles

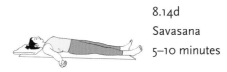

11.7a   11.7b   11.7c

11.1
Rhythmic Breathing
3–4 minutes

11.7d   11.7e   11.7f

III: AFTER PRANAYAMA

8.14d
Savasana
5–10 minutes

15

Irritability, Tension, and Mood Swings: What Your Body Is Saying

PREMENSTRUAL SYNDROME can be defined broadly as recurring physiological, emotional, and behavioral symptoms that occur only before menstruation and are relieved by its onset. Known as PMS, it is estimated to affect 80 to 90 percent of menstruating women, with 10 to 40 percent reporting significant interference with their daily lives.

This chapter offers a sequence of poses to relieve premenstrual emotional symptoms. (Chapter 16 covers migraine headaches, chapter 17 addresses bloating and breast tenderness, and chapter 18 presents solutions to premenstrual insomnia.)

Mood swings that are uncharacteristic of a woman's normal behavior, ranging from grouchiness and irritability to full-blown rage, are often not recognized at the time for what they are—PMS. The emotional upheavals that some women experience during the premenstrual phase can be an amplification of how they feel the rest of the time, especially if they are in the habit of suppressing their feelings or blocking their creativity. A normally mild-mannered woman looks for a fight. Another who is usually confident becomes insecure and unsure of herself. One of my students reports having a very short fuse just before her period; things that she normally would find

mildly upsetting make her weep uncontrollably.

Premenstrual tension may also manifest as hyperactivity and may, in its extreme form, be expressed as paranoia or aggression. For some, premenstrual depression can even precipitate suicide attempts. It takes a lot of yoga and a lot of self-discipline throughout the month to deal with this type of problem, and a woman in this situation should also undergo psychological counseling.

One of the many theories as to the cause of premenstrual mood swings is that estrogen is not being balanced by adequate levels of progesterone. That may be so, but hormone imbalance doesn't happen out of the blue. Menstruation teaches us that we are cyclic beings. The seasons of nature include periods of rest, which promote growth and renewal. The human body is made of the same stuff as the rest of nature and follows similar patterns. When we respect nature's rhythms by, for instance, sleeping when it's dark and waking when it's light, our menstrual cycles are smoother. When we ignore nature's laws, hormones can get out of balance, and we may experience problems during the premenstrual time. When we tune in to our biological rhythms and take some time to rest as menstruation nears, we recognize the true gift of the premenstrual phase:

heightened sensitivity and an enhanced capacity for insight. Ancient cultures knew how to benefit from a woman's sixth sense, which is stronger around the time of menstruation; premenstrual visions were considered sources of wisdom.

This heightened sensitivity is also physical. Dermatologists recommend that a woman refrain from removing unwanted hair (waxing, zapping, tweezing—everything except shaving) in the week before her period, because the skin is more sensitive due to fluctuating hormones. Make sure you get enough rest at this time. Avoid late nights, partying, or working too late at the office. Try not to allow the needs of others overwhelm you in the days leading up to menstruation. Eat regularly, and pay special attention to the foods that you eat. Avoid or cut down on caffeinated drinks. When caffeine intake is heavy and chronic, an allergic reaction can develop that exacerbates PMS symptoms. The caffeine-sensitive woman then tends to reach for more caffeine in order to alleviate the problem, and PMS worsens. (For more information on diet, see chapter 4.)

Practice

Your practice should always take into account your state of mind, your energy level, and where you are in your cycle. The premenstrual phase presents the perfect opportunity to meditate and take stock. Without yoga, the opportunity for transforming chaos into meaning might be thrown away. The sudden venting of pent-up frustrations could cause problems in your relationships and bring pain to your loved ones.

If you are a regular student of yoga, you might notice that as you get close to your period you cannot perform the strenuous postures as well as usual. One of my students reports that she can't hold Chaturanga Dandasana when she is due to

get her period and comes crashing down out of the pose. Other women report that the back bends make them feel nauseous during the premenstrual phase. No two women experience this phase in exactly the same way, so explore for yourself the poses that help you get through or enhance your experience of it.

The following sequence helps to keep mood swings under control. The poses in section I, Supta Baddha Konasana I and Supta Virasana, expand the chest and uplift the heart. They also relieve tiredness. Practice the poses in section II, where the head is supported, to quiet the brain and prepare for the inversions in section III. In section III, Salamba Sirsasana is optional. Those who practice this pose regularly retain a spiritual perspective on life, but if this pose is an effort for you, it may irritate the nerves at this time. Salamba Sarvangasana I is a supported inversion, which alleviates anxiety and dispels irritation. If you have elevated blood pressure, practice Adho Mukha Virasana for 3 minutes before and after Salamba Sirsasana, and Ardha Halasana for 3 minutes before and after Salamba Sarvangasana I. In and of itself, Ardha Halasana has a miraculous capacity to expunge emotional reactivity, including irritability and anger.

By practicing the seated forward bends in section IV, agitation will become tranquility. Mental and emotional turmoil will give way to peace. Janu Sirsasana also helps to normalize blood sugar levels and control food cravings.

For some women, PMS is experienced as confusion, absent-mindedness, restlessness, or a tendency to be accident-prone. The poses in section V, Viparita Karani and Setu Bandha Sarvangasana II, help to stabilize the emotions, provide a deep and profound rest, and promote peace and clarity of mind.

If you are feeling fatigued, begin your practice

with section I. If you are not tired but premenstrual tension has sent your blood pressure soaring (one of the symptoms of which is ringing in the ears), or if you are having difficulty collecting your thoughts or focusing, start instead with section II.

Practice time: 60–90 minutes

I: To Lift Physical Fatigue

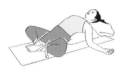

8.2c
Supta Baddha Konasana I
5–10 minutes

8.4c
Supta Virasana
1–2 minutes; increasing to 5 minutes or more with practice

II: To Relieve Mental Strain

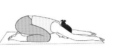

6.10a
Parsva Virasana
10–20 seconds, each side

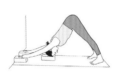

6.9c
Adho Mukha Virasana
30–60 seconds

5.5g
Adho Mukha Svanasana with Head Support
30–60 seconds

5.4h
Uttanasana with Head Support
1 minute

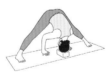

5.15f
Prasarita Padottanasana with Head on Block
1 minute

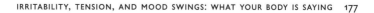

III: To Balance Hormones and Stabilize Emotions

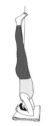

9.2d
Salamba Sirsasana
1–5 minutes, increasing with practice

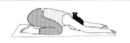

6.9c
Adho Mukha Virasana
30–60 seconds

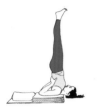

9.3f
Salamba Sarvangasana I
2–5 minutes, increasing to 10 minutes with practice

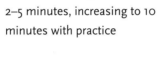

9.8d
Ardha Halasana
5 minutes

IV: To Soothe the Nerves and Calm the Mind

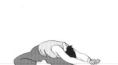

6.12a
Adho Mukha Swastikasana
1–2 minutes,
change cross,
1–2 minutes

7.1f
Janu Sirsasana
30–60 seconds, each side

7.4c
Paschimottanasana
1–5 minutes

V: To Alleviate Anxiety and to Rest

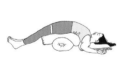

8.10d
Setu Bandha Sarvangasana II
over Crossed Bolsters
3–8 minutes

9.9d
Viparita Karani
5–10 minutes

8.14d
Savasana
5–10 minutes

16

Migraine Headaches
Releasing the Pressure

IGRAINE HEADACHES are three times more common in women than in men and are often triggered by hormonal fluctuations. Women who suffer from migraines often find that the premenstrual phase, when estrogen levels drop just before the onset of bleeding, is a particularly vulnerable time. Others get migraine attacks during menstruation itself. Still others get migraines in the middle of the month, when estrogen levels drop immediately following ovulation.

From the ancient body of knowledge known as ayurveda, we are provided with some profound insights as to why some women are more prone to migraines than others. The human body, like everything else in nature, is made up of five elements: earth, water, fire, air, and space. Out of these five elements arise three distinct patterns that make up three underlying forces, or energy fields, called *doshas*, which pervade the body and the personality.

The three doshas are *kapha*, which is dominated by water and earth and which governs the solid structure of the body; *pitta*, which is dominated by fire and water and which governs the digestive system and bodily heat; and *vata*, which is dominated by air and space and which governs the nervous system and breathing. They all play their part in maintaining health. They also help to shape each person's individual constitution. It is the domination of one over the others that helps us identify our own unique mix of temperament and body type. When we don't pay attention to our health, one or more of the doshas may become weak or aggravated. Then the functions governed by that dosha can become disturbed.

A woman who suffers from migraines is said to have a pitta-influenced cycle. When pitta is balanced, it is the positive energy or heat of the blood. When pitta gets out of control and moves into the cardiovascular system, it affects the blood vessels around the brain. Due to pitta's hot, sharp quality, the cerebral arteries spasm, and the blood vessels in the brain dilate, creating pressure on the nerves and causing a migraine headache.

A woman with a pitta-influenced cycle may also experience loose stools just before or during her period and unusually heavy bleeding. Premenstrually excess pitta creates irritability, pent-up frustration, intense food cravings, excess heat in the body or mind (which in its extreme form results in migraines), acne flare-ups, and other inflammations. Other premenstrual and menstrual symptoms resulting from an excess of pitta energy are vomiting, nausea, and acid stomach.

Chinese medicine also talks about heat and the imbalanced distribution of blood when describing migraine headaches. When the energetic field linked with the liver (liver *chi*) is stagnant, heat accumulates and rises to the head, causing symptoms such as migraines, irritability, and high blood pressure. The head becomes hot and congested, and the hands and feet become cold. The ancient Chinese also understood the connection between pent-up emotions and migraine headache. Once the chi has stopped flowing freely, they say, the result will be emotional imbalance, manifesting as either depression (suppressed liver chi) or irritability (overactive liver chi), or sometimes both. Liver is related to creative energy. Freeing creative energy can often free up congested liver chi and reduce the incidence of migraine headaches.

The liver is of supreme importance to our health and well-being. Artificial hormones, when taken in the form of birth control pills or hormone replacement therapy, place an extra burden on the liver and exacerbate irritability or volatility. Several of my students attributed the sudden flare-up of migraine headaches to the hormones they were taking as part of their fertility treatments.

Occasionally women experience migraine headaches toward the end of or immediately after menstruation. Chinese medicine considers this type of migraine to be caused by a deficiency of blood in the body. Ayurveda and yoga also pay attention to this phase of the cycle (see chapter 13). If you suffer from migraines at the end of your period, slow down and get plenty of rest while you are bleeding. Eat regularly, making sure to consume enough protein to prevent another migraine trigger—low blood sugar. Include blood-nourishing foods in your diet, such as dark green leafy vegetables. Avoid eating heavy meals or eating late. Be mindful of food cravings during the premenstrual phase (see chapter 4). Do not eat too many sweets or carbohydrates, drink coffee or alcohol, or smoke cigarettes, all of which tax the liver.

Practice

Although yoga shares many points of view with ayurveda, it has a somewhat different perspective on the causes of imbalance. According to yoga, the fluctuations of the mind imposing themselves on the body bring about physical and mental imbalance. As such, a focused and committed practice of asana and pranayama is recommended to still the agitated mind (or wake up the dull, sleepy mind), to manage the doshas, and to combat disease.

Practicing a restorative sequence for a few days before you would typically get a migraine will help to stave off an attack. The restorative sequence in chapter 14 followed by extended exhalations (sequence A) and Savasana is a good place to start.

Practice the inverted poses regularly when you are not menstruating. Do some forward bends before and after Salamba Sirsasana to promote calm and quiet brain cells. If you are not ready for Salamba Sirsasana, practice plenty of Adho Mukha Svanasana, Uttanasana, and Prasarita Padottanasana, all with the head supported. Complete your inversions practice with Salamba Sarvangasana, Ardha Halasana (with the eyes closed) to rest the adrenals and also to cool the head, and Setu Bandha Sarvangasana II to calm the nerves. If you are already in the middle of a migraine and your head is pounding, postpone inversions until you feel better.

To maintain healthy liver function, regularly practice the twists, such as Bharadvajasana, Parsva

Virasana, Parsva Swastikasana, Parsva Adho Mukha Swastikasana, and others. (See *Yoga: A Gem for Women,* by Geeta S. Iyengar, for more twists.)

If you are suffering from nausea or acidity, begin with the leaning postures in section I. If you are suffering only from a migraine, begin with the seated forward bends in section II. They help release tension in the back of the neck and shoulders, deflate and cool the blood vessels in the head, and calm the nerves. In particular Janu Sirsasana, Paschimottanasana, and Adho Mukha Virasana produce a cooling effect to the head and help to relieve abdominal tension. Finally, sections III and IV will help you quiet the mind and rest deeply.

Wrap your head (not your eyes) before you start your practice. Make sure that, when you rest your forehead in the forward bends, your eyebrow line remains parallel to the floor, the forehead skin does not get dragged up toward the hairline, and the head does not rest below the shoulders.

Practice time: 60–90 minutes

I: TO RELIEVE NAUSEA, ACIDITY, AND FATIGUE

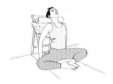

6.2l
Leaning Baddha
Konasana
5–10 minutes

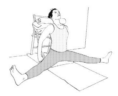

6.3g
Leaning Upavistha
Konasana
5–10 minutes

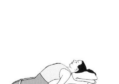

8.4f
Supta Virasana with
Two Bolsters and Blocks
1–2 minutes, with
practice increasing
to 5 or more

II: To Lower Blood Pressure and Relieve Migraine

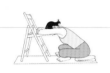

6.9e
Adho Mukha Virasana
with Bolster
30–60 seconds

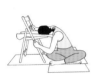

6.12d
Adho Mukha Swastikasana
with Chair
1–2 minutes,
change cross, 1–2 minutes

6.13d
Parsva Adho Mukha
Swastikasana
with Head to Side
20–30 seconds,
change cross of legs,
20–30 seconds

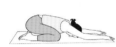

6.9c
Adho Mukha Virasana
30–60 seconds

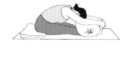

7.4e
Paschimottanasana with
Horizontal Bolster
30 seconds

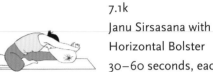

7.1k
Janu Sirsasana with
Horizontal Bolster
30–60 seconds, each side

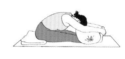

7.4e
Paschimottanasana with
Horizontal Bolster
1–5 minutes

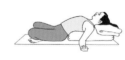

8.6a
Supta Swastikasana
with washcloth
under occipital bone,
at base of skull
2 minutes,
change cross, 2 minutes

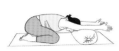

第25贴　反面 凯源-4色-WomandYoga-内页拼版.job

III. To Quiet the Mind

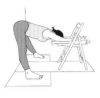

8.10a
Setu Bandha Sarvangasana II
Raise head with a folded
washcloth
3–8 minutes

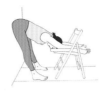

5.4i
Uttanasana with Wall
and Chair
1 minute

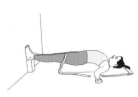

5.15g
Prasarita Padottanasana
with Chair and Wall
1 minute

IV: To Rest

Provided the migraine has abated; if not, repeat
the poses in section II, before ending with Savasana.

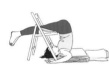

9.8d
Ardha Halasana
Raise head with folded
washcloth
5 minutes

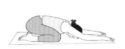

6.9c
Adho Mukha Virasana
30–60 seconds

7.1k
Janu Sirsasana
with Horizontal Bolster
30–60 seconds, each side

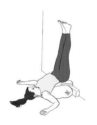

9.9d
Viparita Karani
Raise head with folded
washcloth
5–10 minutes

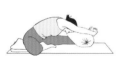

7.4e
Paschimottanasana with
Horizontal Bolster
1–5 minutes

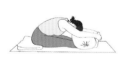

8.10a
Setu Bandha Sarvangasana II
Raise head with
folded washcloth
3–8 minutes

8.14d
Savasana
Raise head with folded
washcloth
5–10 minutes

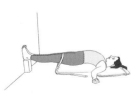

17

Bloating and Breast Tenderness: Easing Symptoms of Congestion

NATURE'S PURPOSE in giving a woman approximately 450 menstrual cycles in the course of her lifetime is not just to discard unfertilized eggs. Every month, menstruation provides her with an opportunity to cleanse and, in the language of ayurveda, to rebalance the *doshas*. Although all three of the doshas (*kapha*, *pitta*, and *vata*) play a vital role in the functioning of the body–mind, it is the dominant dosha that determines your constitutional type. A woman who is predominantly kapha might display the characteristics of physical strength, stability of mind, and courage. However, when kapha energy deteriorates, it can manifest as lethargy, inertia, and sluggishness. If there has been an extra-heavy accumulation of wastes and toxins throughout the month, kapha can backfire during the premenstrual phase, causing congestive symptoms, such as sore and swollen breasts, bloating, and abdominal distention. And you don't have to be kapha-dominant to experience this.

Viewed through the lens of Western medicine, the same symptoms are observed, but from a different perspective. For some women, when the progesterone ratio is low in relation to estrogen, the body cells absorb sodium more readily, which causes excess fluid to be held in the cells. Fluid retention is responsible for a variety of symptoms,

including, heavy and swollen legs, abdominal bloating, puffy hands and feet, joint pain, fatigue, and weight gain. (Premenstrual bloating can increase your body weight anywhere from 1/2 to 5 pounds.) Feelings of heaviness and pressure around the pelvic floor may also occur, due to congestion of the lymph nodes and blood vessels in the area.

Breast problems, ranging from slight swelling to tenderness, that occur during the premenstrual time are usually caused by excess hormonal stimulation. This can arise for several reasons, including an imbalanced lifestyle and chronic stress. One of my students began suffering from painful and swollen breasts when the tension of building her career intensified. She relieved her symptoms by taking herself off to the seashore for a few days each month and by making her yoga practice a priority. (Research has shown that PMS sufferers are less likely to be affected in the summer, suggesting that sunshine or extended hours of daylight supply a hormonal boost).

Many women also suffer from thickening of breast tissue and lumps that come and go. These are usually benign, fluid-filled cysts. Although these can be more prevalent in the days leading to menstruation, anytime you feel a lump in your breast you should have it checked out by your doctor. Other possible causes of lumpiness, cysts, and breast tenderness include having a diet too high in carbohydrates, a deficiency of essential fatty acids, and excess alcohol and caffeine. Coffee and chocolate are the main culprits. A good-quality green tea, however, may be beneficial for the breasts.

In ayurvedic medicine, menstruation is considered an opportunity for cleansing. If we pay attention to diet, stay away from junk food, and practice yoga, stress will lessen and the premenstrual phase will proceed more smoothly.

Practice

The following sequence can help with problems of congestion by stimulating the body's ability to cleanse and purify itself. The reclining poses in section I have a cooling effect on inflamed breast tissue. They also calm the nerves.

When practiced regularly throughout the month, the standing poses in section II keep the abdomen and legs toned, so that when menses comes around, the body is less likely to accumulate fluid. You can practice standing poses during the premenstrual phase (with support if you are feeling tired) to improve circulation.

The sitting poses and twists in sections III and IV squeeze fluid out of the legs, reduce abdominal bloating, and relieve the discomfort of swollen ankles and feet. Baddha Konasana, Upavistha Konasana, and Janu Sirsasana also help keep the genital area free from infection and possible vaginal yeast overgrowth. Raising the arms in all these poses improves circulation in the breasts and helps reduce inflammation.

Many women find their immune systems less robust around this time, causing them to be more prone to infections, such as colds, herpes outbreaks, or an overgrowth of intestinal yeast (which may contribute to abdominal bloating and other premenstrual symptoms). The poses in section V support the immune system. For example, Viparita Dandasana II stimulates circulation in the upper chest and throat and relieves breast tenderness. It also rejuvenates the thymus (located in the upper chest) and tones the abdominal organs, thereby boosting the immune system.

Section VI improves circulation and assist lymph drainage. Salamba Sarvangasana I, Salamba Sarvangasana II, and Halasana and its variations are particularly effective at reducing breast inflammation. They also regulate the glandular system, which in turn regulates the water balance in the body, and they boost immunity.

As a way of addressing the possible psychological component of breast problems, while resting in Savasana, meditate on the concept of receiving. We all deserve love, attention, and fulfillment. As you sink into the pose, allow your muscles to relax and invite the abundant energy from the universe to flow in.

Taken together, the postures that follow have a stabilizing effect emotionally. They reduce mental agitation and calm the nerves.

Practice time: 60–90 minutes

I: To Relieve Fatigue and Breast Tenderness

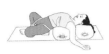

8.3b
Supta Baddha Konasana II
5–10 minutes

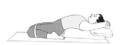

8.4h
Supta Virasana with Arms
above Head
1–5 minutes, increasing with
practice

6.9e
Adho Mukha Virasana with
Bolster
30–60 seconds

II: To Boost Circulation and Reduce Edema

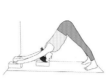

5.5g
Adho Mukha Svanasana with
Head Support
30–60 seconds

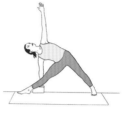

5.9h
Utthita Trikonasana
with Wall and Block
20–30 seconds

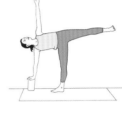

5.11h
Ardha Chandrasana
Against Wall
10–20 seconds

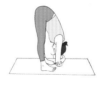

5.4g
Uttanasana with Arms Folded
1 minute

9.2d
Salamba Sirsasana
(continuing practice)
5 minutes, increasing
with practice
or

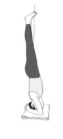

5.15d
Prasarita Padottanasana
(beginning practice)
1 minute

III: To Relieve Tired or Aching Legs and Pelvis and Improve Circulation in the Breasts

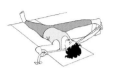

8.13b
Supta Padangustasana II
20–30 seconds, each side

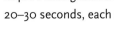

6.8c
Virasana
1–5 minutes

6.10a
Parsva Virasana
20–30 seconds, each side

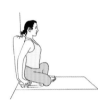

6.8g
Urdhva Baddhangullyasana
in Virasana
10–15 seconds,
change hands, 10–15 seconds

6.2e
Baddha Konasana
Against Wall
with Bolster
1–5 minutes

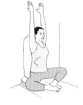

6.2g
Urdhva Hastasana
in Baddha Konasana
10–15 seconds

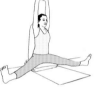

6.3c
Upavistha Konasana
with Wall and Bolster
10–15 seconds

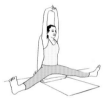

6.3f
Urdhva Baddhangullyasana
in Upavistha Konasana
10–15 seconds, change hands,
10–15 seconds

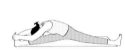

6.4c
Parsva Upavistha Konasana
10–15 seconds, each side

IV: To Reduce Abdominal Bloating

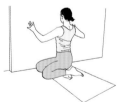

6.15c
Bharadvajasana
30–60 seconds, each side

7.1f
Janu Sirsasana
30–60 seconds, each side

V: To Relieve Painful Breasts and Support the Immune System

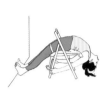

10.2d
Viparita Dandasansa II
(continuing practice)
30–60 seconds,
increasing with practice
or

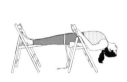

10.2h
Viparita Dandasana II
with Two Chairs
(beginning practice)
30–60 seconds

6.17a
Supported Bharadvajasana II
10–15 seconds, each side

VI: To Soothe Sore, Swollen Breasts and Boost the Immune System

9.3f
Salamba Sarvangasana I
2–5 minutes, increasing with
practice
Tired or cannot hold for long:
practice with support

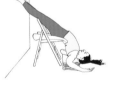

9.4e
Salamba Sarvangasana II
3–5 minutes, or more

9.6b
Halasana
1–5 minutes

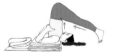

9.6g
Supta Konasana
30–60 seconds

9.7a
Parsva Halasana
10–20 seconds, each side

9.8e
Ardha Halasana with Thighs
Raised on Bolster
5 minutes

8.10d
Setu Bandha Sarvangasana II
over Crossed Bolsters
3–8 minutes

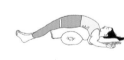

9.9d
Viparita Karani
5–10 minutes

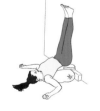

8.14g
Savasana with Upper Back
Supported
5–10 minutes

第27贴　正面　凯源-4色-WomandYoga-内页拼版.job

18

Insomnia: Calming the Nerves and Inducing Sleep

ACH WOMAN experiences the phases of the menstrual cycle in her own unique way. But one experience seems to be universal: cyclic sleep disturbances. It is when hormone levels fluctuate the most rapidly (such as during the late luteal phase, from around days 25 to 28, when hormone levels drop markedly) that women notice the most disrupted mood and sleep patterns. A student of mine feels like she's taken speed during this phase, almost as if she is shaking inside. As soon as she gets her period, she settles down and her sleep returns to normal.

The connection between hormonal fluctuations and insomnia is borne out by the National Sleep Foundation's Women and Sleep Study, conducted in 1998. Over 71 percent of the women polled reported that their sleep was disturbed by symptoms associated with menstruation. The most commonly reported cause of disturbed sleep was bloating, followed closely by other factors, including cramping, headaches, and tender breasts. And proving that not all women react to monthly hormonal fluctuations in the same way, 28 percent of women polled reported that they sleep more at this time.

The study also reports that the average woman sleeps only 6 hours and 41 minutes a night during the working week. Prevailing wisdom has it that we must sleep for at least 8 or 9 hours for optimum health. But the latest findings suggest that we may do better with less rather than more sleep. A Japanese study published by the London Sleep Center shows that a person's mortality risk increases for every hour they sleep more than seven and a half. Indeed, the best survival rate is experienced by those who sleep between six and a half and seven and a half hours a night on weekdays.

So how do you know whether you are getting enough sleep? First ask yourself, How do I feel? If you feel tired all the time, it may be that your individual sleep requirement is not being met. However, it may be that *when* you sleep is just as important to your health and well-being as how long you sleep. Studies have shown that our systems do the majority of their recharging and repairing between the hours of 11 P.M. and 1 A.M., which is when the gall bladder dumps its toxins. If you are awake during these hours, the toxins back up into the liver, which overloads the system and erodes health. This sets up a negative cycle for the menstruating woman, further stressing the body's defense systems and putting them at risk for disease and emotional disturbance.

Of course, something else happens when we don't sleep: we don't dream. And dream deprivation is every bit as responsible for physical and emotional distress as sleep deprivation. In fact, the symptoms of dream deprivation—irritability, depression, and lethargy—are very similar to those of premenstrual tension. And premenstrual symptoms increase when a woman's sleep is disturbed and are less when she gets the sleep she needs.

Ayurvedic wisdom agrees with current scientific studies that the body is cleansed during the first half of the night, but it goes one step further, telling us that the subtle body is cleansed during the second half of the night. The process known as rapid eye movement (REM) signifies that the brain is active, and through the process of dreaming it is discharging, or in some way processing, our experiences so that when we awaken the mind is clean and clear and ready for the new day. This is particularly important for women; toward the end of the cycle, from around day 25, the length of time spent dreaming increases.

According to Iyengar Yoga, dreams fall into three categories: symbolic dreams that require interpretation, obsessive dreams born out of fear or caused by a chemical imbalance of the *doshas*, and revelatory dreams that transmit metaphysical concepts. This last kind of dream, where spiritual ideas come through from the unconscious mind, has always played a vital role for mystics and yogis. Similarly a woman whose yoga practice is established may find that her dreams are a source of inspiration, particularly during the premenstrual phase. Just as certain tribal women had access to divine knowledge around this time, modern women may find that the premenstrual dream boosts their creativity. As some abilities diminish during this time, such as concentration and the ability to think logically, other areas, such as the ability to free-associate, may open up.

A simple and effective way to maintain health and longevity is to rise at the same time every morning, with the sun if possible, and to go to bed early, around 10 or 11 o'clock. Other pointers to getting a good night's sleep include eating a balanced diet, not eating too late in the evening, and avoiding caffeine and alcohol. Try to sleep in complete darkness; having any kind of light entering in your bedroom disturbs the body's natural circadian rhythms. Finally, if you like to read before drifting off to sleep, read something spiritual.

Many studies have shown that exercise can help alleviate depression and insomnia. In my experience, yoga is more effective than exercise when it comes to dealing with sleep disturbances. But you don't have to wait until your period comes around to practice yoga. Make it a part of your life. Practice yoga consistently throughout the month so that premenstrual problems don't overwhelm you or disturb your work and relationships.

Practice

A regular and challenging yoga practice that includes standing poses (see chapter 5) and back bends (see chapter 10) relieves tension and burns off negative nervous energy. It is also much easier to sleep when you have had a good workout. It is best to practice the energetic postures early in the day and the inversions later on. If that is hard to manage, a short practice that incorporates both, practiced at any time of the day, will have a profound, positive effect.

During the premenstrual phase, however, is not a good time to do a challenging yoga practice. A student of mine reports that she gets shaky if she practices back bends when she's close to her period. Other women experience nausea when practicing back bends at this time. The sequence that follows does contain a back bend: Viparita Dandasana I, which is supported, so it will not overstimulate your nervous or digestive systems. If it does, however, skip it and move on to the next pose. This pose helps reduce glandular stress and frees up the breath.

The inversions, such as Salamba Sirsasana, Salamba Sarvangasana II, and Halasana, along with Setu Bandha Sarvangasana II over Crossed Bolsters, promote healthy and peaceful sleep, but omit them if you are practicing this sequence during menstruation.

The seated forward bends help pacify the brain, calm the nerves, and quell anxiety. Practice them with the emphasis on resting the forehead. Pass briefly through the first stage, with the head up, in Janu Sirsasana and Paschimottanasana. Stay for as long as you can with the head down and the torso and chest extended.

You can also practice pranayama to soothe the nervous system and calm a restless and agitated mind. For premenstrual or menstrual insomnia, focus on extending the exhalations (see sequence A in chapter 14).

Remember, this is a premenstrual sequence. If you have insomnia and want to practice it during your period, omit the inversions. If you practice in the evening, do it before your (light) evening meal.

You can practice with the head wrapped in all of the poses, to help you stay quiet and to reduce mental activity.

Practice time: 60–90 minutes

I: To Remove Fatigue and Nervous Energy

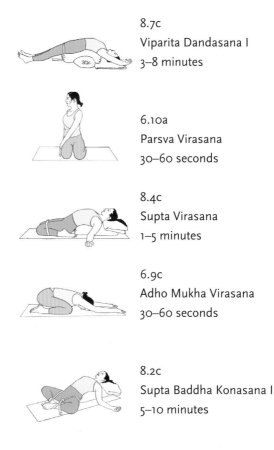

8.7c
Viparita Dandasana I
3–8 minutes

6.10a
Parsva Virasana
30–60 seconds

8.4c
Supta Virasana
1–5 minutes

6.9c
Adho Mukha Virasana
30–60 seconds

8.2c
Supta Baddha Konasana I
5–10 minutes

II: To Rest the Heart and Quiet the Mind

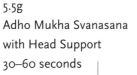

5.5g
Adho Mukha Svanasana
with Head Support
30–60 seconds

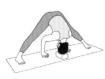

5.4h
Uttanasana
with Head Support
1 minute

5.15f
Prasarita Padottanasana
with Head on Block
1 minute

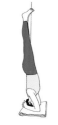

9.2d
Salamba Sirsasana
(continuing practice)
1–5 minutes, increasing
with practice
or

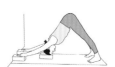

5.5g
Adho Mukha Svanasana
with Head Support
(beginning practice)
30–60 seconds

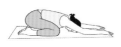

6.9c
Adho Mukha Virasana
30–60 seconds

III: To Rest the Brain and Relieve Tension

10.2d
Viparita Dandasana II
30–60 seconds, increasing
to 5 minutes with practice

or, if practicing during
menstruation

10.2i
Viparita Dandasana II with
Head and Feet Supported
30–60 seconds, increasing
to 5 minutes with practice

6.17a
Supported Bharadvajasana II
20–30 seconds, each side

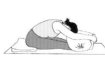

7.4e
Paschimottanasana
with Horizontal Bolster
20–30 seconds

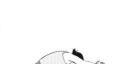

7.1k
Janu Sirsasana
with Horizontal Bolster
20–30 seconds

6.12a
Adho Mukha Swastikasana
30–60 seconds,
change cross,
30–60 seconds

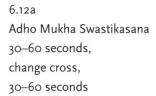

7.4e
Paschimottanasana
with Horizontal Bolster
3–5 minutes

IV: To Stabilize Hormonal Activity and Promote Peace Within

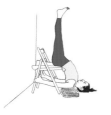

9.4e
Salamba Sarvangasana II
2–5 minutes

9.4f
Viparita Karani in Salamba
Sarvangasana II
30–60 seconds

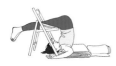

9.4g
Baddha Konasana in Salamba
Sarvangasana II
30–60 seconds

9.8d
Ardha Halasana
3–5 minutes

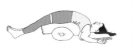

8.10d
Setu Bandha Sarvangasana II
over Crossed Bolsters
3–8 minutes

V: To Rest

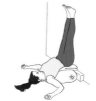

9.9d
Viparita Karani
5–10 minutes

8.14g
Savasana with Upper Back
Supported
5–10 minutes

19
Abdominal Cramps and Low Back Pain: Soothing Poses

AN ASTONISHING 60 percent of all women are reported to experience menstrual cramps at some point during their reproductive years. While this obviously common occurrence may be more prevalent in modern industrialized societies, evidence has filtered down to us from the past that suggests that menstrual cramps are not a new invention. From a recent study on the medicinal properties of cannabis, we learn that as far back as the seventh century B.C.E in ancient Mesopotamia, and continuing across continents and cultures, women have suffered from menstrual cramps (or dysmenorrhea). Even Queen Victoria of England, it seems, was prone to them and was prescribed cannabis to relieve her monthly pains. But only in the last two decades have menstrual cramps been considered worthy of serious investigation by the medical profession.

Menstrual cramping is divided into two types: primary and secondary. Primary dysmenorrhea, which most women suffer from, is not caused by disease. The excessive release of prostaglandins (a protein that is also triggered to bring on labor) aids the rhythmic (and sometimes painful) movement of the uterus needed to help expel the endometrial lining. Expelling a blood clot from the uterus—a normal part of menstruation for some women—can also cause a spasm of pain,

which can vary from mild twinges to extreme spasmodic contractions. This type of dysmenorrhea usually becomes less painful as a woman ages and may stop entirely after she has a baby. Secondary dysmenorrhea is a consequence of an underlying problem, most commonly endometriosis. Other causes include pelvic infection, irritation from an intrauterine device, fibroids, or ovarian cysts. Cervical stenosis (a narrowing of the cervix due to scar tissue) can also cause menstrual cramps. If you suffer from severe cramping, it is imperative that you seek medical advice to find out if there is any disease involved.

Menstrual cramps can also send pain waves through the groins, down the legs, and into the lower back. Spasms may stimulate the intestines and bladder and produce symptoms of nausea, vomiting, diarrhea, and frequent urination. Cramping may also trigger migraine headaches.

Ayurvedic physicians recommend that women pay particular attention to diet in the week leading up to menstruation. Those prone to cramping are advised to avoid foods that constipate. Rosita Arvigo and Nadine Epstein, in their book *Rainforest Home Remedies*, pass along the Mayan view that dysmenorrhea is often caused by a prolapsed uterus that is not able to flush itself out completely from month to month. Eventually the buildup of congested blood in the uterus causes painful periods, as the body uses more force to try to eliminate the material. They recommend massage to return the uterus to its proper position and to strengthen the ligaments that hold it in place.

B. K. S. Iyengar recommends including Virabhadrasana I into your regular practice to ensure that the pelvic and uterine muscles remain strong and the uterus stays in its proper position. When the uterus is prolapsed as well as displaced, it is recommended to practice Salamba Sirsasana and Salamba Sarvangasana I to help move the uterus away from the pelvic floor. Back bends, such as Ustrasana, Viparita Dandasana II, Urdhva Dhanurasana, and Supta Virasana, are also recommended to prevent and correct a displaced uterus.

When dysmenorrhea is caused by endometriosis, cramping can be severe and debilitating. Endometriosis is a condition in which tissue from the lining of the uterus (the endometrium) migrates to other parts of the pelvis, implants itself onto other organs, and bleeds internally along with menstruation. There are many theories about the causes of endometriosis. Reflux menstruation, where the menstrual flow gets backed up and out of the fallopian tubes into the abdominal cavity, is a common enough occurrence. But all women show some retrograde bleeding, and not all women develop a condition where endometrial fragments fix onto internal pelvic organs. One theory is that endometriosis is the result of a dysfunctional immune system. A healthy immune system should destroy this renegade tissue, but when it is too weak to react, the tissue begins to grow. Systemic yeast (Candida), which often flourishes when the immune system is weak, has been associated with endometriosis. Because the exact cause for endometriosis remains unknown, our best approach is to go for whole body–mind health, to encourage healing.

Menstrual pain is often related to emotional pain. Some clinicians cite emotional stress as a contributing factor in endometriosis, which they consider to be an estrogen-dominant condition. When stress causes the adrenal glands to become dysfunctional, hormone levels are no longer held in balance, and estrogen levels soar.

Stress can also cause the abdominal muscles to become hard and tense, and this can contribute to menstrual cramps, as well as to other menstrual problems. B. K. S. Iyengar recommends a regular practice of back bends (*not to be practiced when cramping is actually occurring*) to create elasticity and strength in the pelvic muscles and help prevent menstrual cramping. A woman's creative center is her uterus, and it works like a sense organ. Raw and responsive, it reacts to negative emotions and upset. Gynecologist Marcel Pick told me that, in her medical practice, women with severe and chronic menstrual cramping often have unfinished family issues, such as a history of sexual abuse, an overcontrolling father, problems with a partner, or alcoholism in the family.

So what can we do about menstrual discomfort? Understanding the cycle of cause and effect helps, but not enough to alleviate monthly pains. Start by learning to set boundaries in your personal life and at work. Make sure you get sufficient rest and quiet time while menstruating. Experience shows us that menstrual cramps can be controlled to some degree by improving your diet (see chapter 4). A study of Italian women found that the risk of endometriosis dropped by 40 percent when women ate more green vegetables and fruit. Those who ate large amounts of red meat increased their risk between 8 and 100 percent.

A balanced yoga practice can help on many levels. It strengthens us mentally, so we are better able to deal with life's problems. As a consequence, we are less likely to hold mental anguish in the tissues of the body. It can also release the imprint of past trauma on the body. Yoga asana and pranayama calm the adrenals and the nerves, restore hormone balance, relax the abdominal muscles, and stimulate circulation within the pelvis, all of which go a long way toward eliminating menstrual cramps.

Practice

No two women experience menstrual pain in the same way, so read these notes carefully. Select the sections appropriate to your symptoms (whether they be low back pain, abdominal cramping, or both) from the following sequence.

The standing poses in sections I and II are optional. Some women may be too tired to practice them; others may feel worse if they don't stretch. Uttitha Trikonasana Facing the Wall and Ardha Chandrasana Facing the Wall can relieve both abdominal cramps and low back pain. Make sure you move the sacrum well in, so the lower abdomen gets extended. Women tend to hold the uterus in as a reaction to stressful situations, and then it becomes a habit, so make sure you don't strain or grip the abdominal area, particularly during menstruation, and don't stay in these two poses more than 20 seconds on each side. Supta Padangustasana II can also relieve menstrual cramping.

The three standing forward bends in section II, Uttanasana, Adho Mukha Svanasana, and Prasarita Padottanasana with Chair and Wall, can also alleviate menstrual pain, particularly when it is experienced in the lower back. They also rest the brain.

The postures in section III are recommended by Geeta Iyengar to relieve cramping *only* when is caused by endometriosis. They also help relieve

nausea. (If you suffer from endometriosis, consult an experienced teacher for the best way to practice throughout the remainder of the month).

Whether menstrual cramps are caused by endometriosis or not, continue with the reclining poses in section IV. They calm the nerves and release the tense muscles and blocked circulation that may be contributing to abdominal spasms. These postures also help relieve diarrhea.

Those with endometriosis should skip section V and finish up with section VI, to cool down and rest.

However, if you have fibroids or cysts, or if you are experiencing fatigue in your thighs, *begin* your practice with section IV to reduce abdominal heaviness and relax the pelvic area. Continue with the standing poses in sections I and II if you wish, to further reduce cramping and to boost energy.

The seated forward bends, in which the belly is supported, follow in section V. They soothe the abdomen, but they are especially effective in relieving low back pain and providing relief from the stress of menstruation. Decide for yourself whether a horizontal or vertical bolster works best to relieve your symptoms. Do whatever is easiest on your spine and most soothing for your head and back. Most important, make sure the abdomen is not constricted. If these forward bends make abdominal cramping worse, discontinue them for the time being. Pick them up again when your menstrual cycle is over or at such time when cramps are not an issue.

Parsva Adho Mukha Swastikasana can relieve burning sensations in the lower back. Most twists are not practiced during menstruation because the squeezing and turning of the waist and belly tends to overexcite the system at this time and cause the menstrual flow to be heavier. However, in this twist, which is combined with a forward bend, focus on soothing pain in the lower back, rather than on a strong rotation of the spine. Have plenty of support under your head.

The poses in section VI will restore the nerves and help you to rest deeply.

Practice time: 60–90 minutes

I: To Boost Energy and Relieve Menstrual Cramps

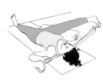

8.13c
Supta Padangusthasana
II with Bolster
20–30 seconds, each side

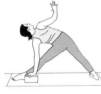

5.9i Utthita Trikonasana
Facing Wall
15–20 seconds, each side

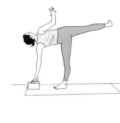

5.11j
Ardha Chandrasana
Facing Wall
15–20 seconds, each side
or

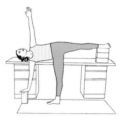

5.11g
Ardha Chandrasana with
Leg Support
15–20 seconds, each side

II: To Relieve Low Back Pain and Rest the Brain

5.4h
Uttanasana with Head
Support (turn toes in)
1 minute
or

5.4i
Uttanasana
with Wall and Chair
1 minute

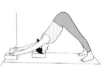

5.5g
Adho Mukha Svanasana with
Head Support
30–60 seconds

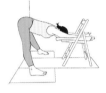

5.15g
Prasarita Padottanasana with
Chair and Wall
1 minute

III: When Menstrual Cramps Are Caused by Endometriosis

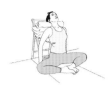

6.2l
Leaning Baddha Konasana
1–5 minutes

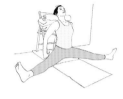

6.3g
Leaning Upavistha Konasana
1–2 minutes

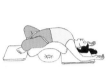

8.11b
Supta Baddha Konasana
in Viparita Dandasana II
1–5 minutes

IV: To Reduce Abdominal Tension and Fatigue in the Thighs and Relieve Cramps

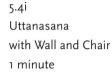

8.3b
Supta Baddha Konasana II
5–10 minutes

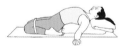

8.4c
Supta Virasana
1–5 minutes, increasing
with practice

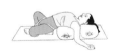

8.5g
Matsyasana with Blanket Roll
30–60 seconds or more,
change cross, 30–60 seconds
or more
or

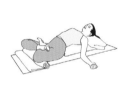

8.6b
Supta Swastikasana
with Blankets
1–2 minutes, change cross,
1–2 minutes

V: To Reduce Low Back Pain and Relieve Stress

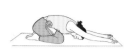

6.9f
Adho Mukha Virasana with Blanket Roll
30–60 seconds

6.10a
Parsva Virasana
30–60 seconds, each side

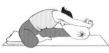

7.1k
Janu Sirsasana with Horizontal Bolster
30–60 seconds, each side
or

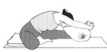

7.1l
Janu Sirsasana with Vertical Bolster and Blankets
30–60 seconds, each side

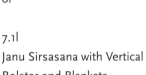

6.3a
Upavistha Konasana
10–15 seconds

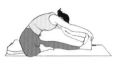

6.4d
Parsva Upavistha Konasana with Bolster
30–60 seconds, each side

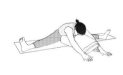

6.5c
Adho Mukha Upavistha Konasana with Bolster and Blanket
30–60 seconds

6.2i
Adho Mukha Baddha Konasana with Wall and Bolster
1 minute

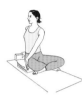

6.11c
Parsva Swastikasana
30–60 seconds, change cross, 30–60 seconds

6.13b or 6.13c
Parsva Adho Mukha Swastikasana
30–60 seconds, change cross of legs, 30–60 seconds

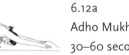

6.12a
Adho Mukha Swastikasana
30–60 seconds

VI: To Restore the Nerves and Rest

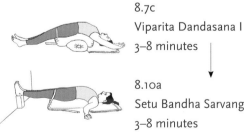

8.7c
Viparita Dandasana I
3–8 minutes

8.10a
Setu Bandha Sarvangasana II
3–8 minutes

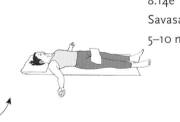

8.14e
Savasana with Sandbag
5–10 minutes

20

Excessive and Prolonged Bleeding:
Stabilizing the System

EXCESSIVE BLEEDING (menorrhagia) is considered to be bleeding that soaks a sanitary napkin or tampon every hour or so. Prolonged bleeding (also menorrhagia) refers to periods that go on for longer than seven days. Most women have a heavy period at some time in their lives and more often than not, the system rights itself by the next period. If it does not, you should get a medical check-up.

The most common cause for excessive or prolonged menstrual bleeding is the erratic production of hormones and a cycle that has not been preceded by ovulation. The follicle may ripen but fail to rupture and the ovum is not released. Since it is the empty follicle that excretes progesterone, progesterone comes to a halt. The cycle continues as usual, but the uterus cannot stop its bleeding properly without supplies of progesterone. Dropped progesterone levels occur more often during peri-menopause (the years leading up to menopause).

A heavy or irregular menstrual flow is also common in adolescence. In both these phases, hormonal activity is transforming for the next stage of life, and the normal pattern of progesterone and estrogen production is imbalanced.

Excessive menstrual bleeding may also be caused by stress. The woman who does not know how to set boundaries and keeps pouring out her energy may also have a tendency to bleed heavily. According to ayurvedic wisdom, excessive menstrual bleeding is common among women who have a high *pitta* (fire) constitution; unresolved anger, resentment, or hostility can throw this *dosha* out of balance.

Endometriosis, which may also cause cysts and scar tissue to form around the ovary, can also disrupt ovarian function.

Excessive and prolonged bleeding may also be the result of an infection caused by an intrauterine device (IUD), blocked fallopian tubes, endometrial polyps, or cervical erosion. This condition can also indicate cancer or pelvic infections.

Another fairly common cause of excessive bleeding is the presence of fibroid tumors embedded on the inside walls of the uterus. There are many theories as to the cause of fibroid tumors (which remarkably 75 to 80 percent of all women are found to have by the time they die). One theory is that underlying emotions such as feelings of emptiness, loneliness, and unfulfilled creativity may result in the hormonal imbalance that triggers their growth. Some researchers have suggested that fibroids, like endometriosis, may be linked to an overgrowth of Candida yeast or allergies.

Another theory is that chronic abdominal tension, or aggressive exercise where the uterus is continually and repeatedly tensed, may exacerbate fibroid growth. Tampon use has also been suspected as a contributing factor. All of these conditions tend to thrive when estrogen is not balanced by progesterone.

Artificial estrogen, such as that found in birth control pills, may speed up fibroid growth. It is also known that fibroids (as well as endometriosis) runs in families, although it is becoming clear that the genetic predisposition to disease can be counteracted by modifying one's diet and practicing yoga.

In the absence of any substantial research on the subject of menorrhagia, we have to take charge of our own bodies. For some reason, the immune system has been compromised and nutritional deficiencies as well as tension could be contributing factors.

Practice

When a profuse or prolonged menstrual flow results in anemia or exhaustion, do not do allow your regular yoga practice (the one that you do when you are not menstruating) to further deplete your energy. Go easy on the standing poses. (Note: Sequence A does not include standing poses and Sequence B does.) Avoid jumping between poses. Avoid the unsupported back bends, or indeed anything that may stress or irritate the system. Those with endometriosis should seek the advice of a qualified teacher for which asanas to perform (and how to perform them) during the rest of the month.

The reclining poses are particularly important if you have a tendency to bleed heavily. Practice Supta Baddha Konasana, Supta Virasana, Supta Swastikasana, Setu Bandha Sarvangasana, and Supta Baddha Konasana in Setu Bandha Sarvangasana regularly, throughout the month, to restore energy and relax the abdominal organs.

Practice sequences A and B regularly, between periods, to eventually free yourself from the problem of an excessively heavy flow. Practice sequence C during menstruation to rebalance and rest.

When your period finishes, practice the postmenstrual sequence in chapter 13. If an excessively heavy flow has left you really depleted, begin the recovery postmenstrual sequence with Savasana with Sandbag, Supta Baddha Konasana, and Supta Virasana.

Sequence A: Regular Practice

Practice Upavista Konasana, Baddha Konasana, Padmasana, Matsyasana in sections I and II to improve circulation throughout the pelvis and align the pelvic organs. The inverted poses in section III quiet the mind, stabilize hormonal output, and also help regulate the flow.

Prolonged bleeding causes tension, and tension causes prolonged bleeding; practice the seated forward bends in section IV to alleviate abdominal tension, take the pressure off the brain, and produce your own progesterone. Practice them with adequate support, so the abdomen is not constricted. Sit on a stack of blankets to relax the belly, and rest your head on a bolster or chair. Finally, practice the poses in section V to reduce flow and rest.

Practice time: 60–90 minutes

I: To Tone Reproductive Organs and Regularize Menstrual Flow

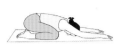

6.9c
Adho Mukha Virasana
30–60 seconds

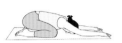

5.5g
Adho Mukha Svanasana
with Head Support
30–60 seconds

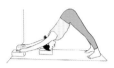

6.9c
Adho Mukha Virasana
10–20 seconds

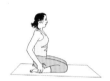

6.8c
Virasana
1–5 minutes

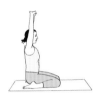

6.8g
Urdhva Baddangullyasana in
Virasana
10–20 seconds, each side

6.3c
Upavistha Konasana
with Wall and Bolster
30–60 seconds

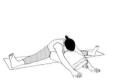

6.3e
Urdhva Hastasana in
Upavistha Konasana
10–15 seconds

6.5c
Adho Mukha Upavistha
Konasana with Bolster
and Blanket
30–60 seconds

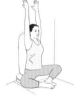

6.2e
Baddha Konasana
Against Wall with Bolster
1–5 minutes

6.2g
Urdhva Hastasana
in Baddha Konasana
10–15 seconds

6.2i
Adho Mukha Baddha
Konasana with Wall
and Bolster
30–60 seconds

II: To Release Pelvic Tension and Promote Flexibility in Hip Joints

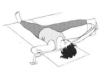

8.13b
Supta Padangusthasana II
with Bolster
20–30 seconds, each side

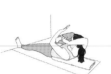

6.14c
Supta Padangustasana III
20 seconds, each side

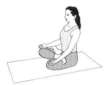

6.14i
Padmasana
20–30 seconds, each side

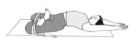

8.5e
Matsyasana
1–3 minutes, change cross,
1–3 minutes

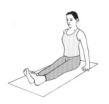

6.1a
Dandasana
20–30 seconds

III: To Improve the Function of the Glandular System and Align the Pelvic Organs

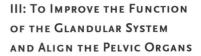

5.4h
Uttanasana with Head
Support
1 minute

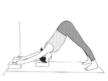

5.5g
Adho Mukha Svanasana
with Head Support
30–60 seconds

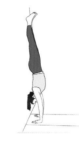

9.1d
Adho Mukha Vrksasana
20–30 seconds

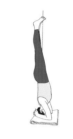

9.2d
Salamba Sirsasana
(continuing practice)
1–5 minutes, increasing
with practice

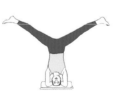

9.2g
Upavistha Konasana
in Salamba Sirsasana
(continuing practice)
15–20 seconds

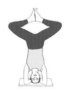

9.2h
Baddha Konasana
in Salamba Sirsasana
(continuing practice)
15–20 seconds

or

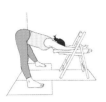

5.15g
Prasarita Padottanasana
with Chair and Wall
(beginning practice)
1–2 minutes

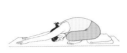

6.12a
Adho Mukha Swastikasana
20–30 seconds, each side

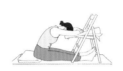

7.4h
Paschimottanasana with
Legs Apart and Chair
20–30 seconds

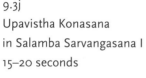

9.3f
Salamba Sarvangasana I
3–5 minutes, increasing
with practice

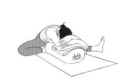

7.1m
Janu Sirsasana
with Legs Apart
30–60 seconds, each side

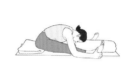

9.3j
Upavistha Konasana
in Salamba Sarvangasana I
15–20 seconds

7.4g
Paschimottanasana with
Legs Apart and Bolster
3–5 minutes

9.3k
Baddha Konasana
in Salamba Sarvangasana I
15–20 seconds

V: TO REST

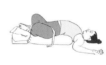

8.11c
Supta Baddha Konasana in
Setu Bandhasana
3–8 minutes

9.6b
Halasana
30–60 seconds

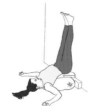

9.9d
Viparita Karani
5–10 minutes

9.6g
Supta Konasana
15–20 seconds

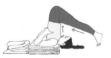

8.14e
Savasana with Sandbag
5–10 minutes

Sequence B:
Adding Standing Poses to Regular Practice

When you are feeling stronger, you can add standing poses to sequence A. Omit sections I and II and begin with section III. Add these two standing poses after Adho Mukha Svanasana, and continue with the remainder of sequence A.

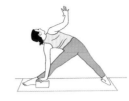

5.9i
Utthita Trikonasana
Facing Wall
30-60 seconds, each side

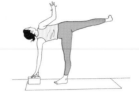

5.11j
Ardha Chandrasana
Facing Wall
30-60 seconds, each side

Sequence C:
Practice During Menstruation

Practice sequence C during menstruation to rebalance and rest. These postures help reduce fatigue and an excessively heavy flow. They can also be practiced during the heavy phase of your period (most women experience a heavier flow for one or two days during their period and this is perfectly normal). Later on in your period, when the flow becomes lighter, practice one of the other menstrual sequences in this book. The poses in this sequence soothe the nerves, relieve pelvic soreness, lessen diarrhea, and ease discomfort. They are appropriate for women whose excessive bleeding is brought on by menopause, stress, endometriosis, fibroids, or any other organic cause, because there is nothing here that would irritate or heat the system, and they will help to stem the flow. Make sure your abdomen and throat are relaxed throughout your practice.

Everyone can start with section I. If excessive or prolonged bleeding is caused by endometriosis, then also practice the poses in section II. If it is not caused by endometriosis, omit section II.

Everyone can continue with section III. Ardha Chandrasana with Leg Support often works when nothing else does, to reduce an excessively heavy menstrual flow. Everyone should finish with section IV, to rest.

When your body detects that too much blood is being lost, your blood pressure may drop as a protective mechanism, and you may get cold. Do not practice in a draft, and have a blanket ready in case you need it.

Practice time: 60–90 minutes

I: FOR EXCESSIVE AND PROLONGED FLOW: SOME COOLING POSES

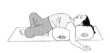

8.13c
Supta Padangustasana II
with Bolster
20–30 seconds, each side

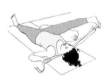

8.3b
Supta Baddha Konasana II
5–10 minutes

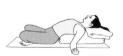

8.6a
Supta Swastikasana
2 minutes, change cross,
2 minutes

II: FOR ENDOMETRIOSIS: TO CREATE SPACE IN THE LOWER ABDOMEN

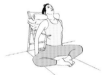

6.2l
Leaning Baddha Konasana
1–5 minutes

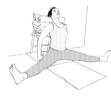

6.3g
Leaning Upavistha Konasana
1–2 minutes

8.8a
Supta Baddha Konasana
in Viparita Dandasana I
2–5 minutes

III: To Regularize Menstrual Flow and Relieve Tension

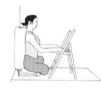

6.2f
Baddha Konasana
Against Wall with Chair
1–5 minutes

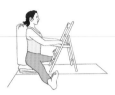

6.3d
Upavistha Konasana
Wall, Bolster, and Chair
1–2 minutes

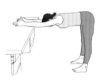

6.5c
Adho Mukha Upavistha
Konasana with Bolster
and Blanket
30–60 seconds

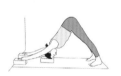

5.4j
Uttanasana with Arms
on Countertop or Chair
1 minute

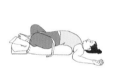

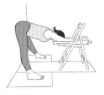

5.5g
Adho Mukha Svanasana
with Head Support
30 seconds

5.15g
Prasarita Padottanasana
with Chair and Wall
1 minute

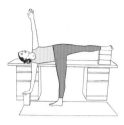

5.11g
Ardha Chandrasana
with Leg Support
15–20 seconds, each side

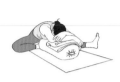

7.1m
Janu Sirsasana
with Legs Apart
20–30 seconds, each side

IV: To Reduce the Flow and Rest

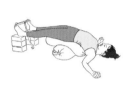

8.10f
Setu Bandha Sarvangasana II
over Crossed Bolsters with
Blocks, Legs Apart
3–5 minutes

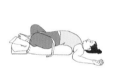

8.11c
Supta Baddha Konasana
in Setu Bandhasana
1–3 minutes

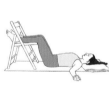

8.14f
Savasana with Legs
Supported on Chair
5–10 minutes

21

Scanty Periods: Strengthening the System

Hypomenorrhea refers to a scanty menstrual flow that lasts only a day or two. It is often accompanied by cramps, a tense and rigid abdomen, and constipation (sometimes alternating with loose stools). (See chapter 19, for how to relieve these symptoms during menstruation). The cycle can be regular or irregular, although the spacing between periods can often be longer than a month.

The menstrual cycle is an indicator of your overall energetic balance. If you have scanty periods, it is worth checking out your general health, because hypomenorrhea is often indicative of depletion. One theory has it that the body shuts down menstrual function during stressful times in order to prevent pregnancy during times of turmoil. If you wear yourself out, either by overworking, overexercising, or simply by burning the candle at both ends, you may find that over time your periods get lighter. Women who suffer from a distorted body image and are obsessed with staying thin (and either starve themselves or overexercise, or both) often experience a reduced menstrual flow. A woman who is hooked on running and whose periods have gotten lighter to the point where she is just spotting may find that her periods may stop altogether.

Scanty periods can also occur when inner tensions disturb hormone balance, disrupting the mechanisms that create a healthy menstrual flow. Anxiety and stress can create tension in the diaphragm and lower abdomen, which may obstruct the internal pathways (controlled by *apana vayu*, the energy that governs downward movement) through which lymph and blood flow. The consequent lack of nourishment to the reproductive organs may result in a very light period and, in some cases, pain, discomfort, or disease, such as pelvic inflammatory disease.

Apana vayu's downward course can also be impaired by constipation, which could be the result of a rich or mucus-producing diet, a sedentary lifestyle, stress, or a combination of all three.

From a Western medical perspective, constipation can be exacerbated by hormonal imbalance. The function of progesterone is to relax the smooth muscles of the uterus during pregnancy so it will not contract and expel the fetus. High levels of progesterone during the second half of the month can cause decreased movement in the intestines and slow down the digestion of food, increasing the likelihood of constipation. When menstruation begins, the uterus shrinks to its normal size, easing the restriction on the colon. While the initial stool can be hard, it may be followed by diarrhea.

A light menstrual flow can also be due to underdevelopment of the uterus or deficiency in the formation of the ovaries or endocrine glands. Young girls sometimes have very light periods, although this usually corrects itself with time. Women in perimenopause (around the beginning of menopause) often experience lighter periods. (They also sometimes experience very heavy and irregular periods).

The use of birth control pills often causes scanty periods. An ovarian cyst can sometimes lead to more frequent and lighter bleeding than normal. Short or scanty periods may also be the result of either hypothyroidism or hyperthyroidism, where the thyroid gland is not working properly.

When the desire to be thin crosses the boundary from healthy self-discipline to obsessive-compulsive behavior (such as bulimia) that interferes with your menstrual cycle, then consider what you are doing and take some steps to establish a measure of balance. There are several things you can do to restore a healthy menstrual flow: eat the foods that make you vitally healthy, maintain regular sleeping habits, and replace an unhealthy exercise program with yoga.

Practice

If you are seriously underweight or exhausted, practice the restorative sequences given in chapters 15 and 16. When you are ready for a stronger practice (when you have put on a little weight and are not so fatigued), start by building strength slowly. Very thin women often have bad posture due to weakness, and it may be an effort for them to stand upright. They may also be suffering from bone loss. Bones get stronger when you learn to control your muscles. For instance, when you draw the quadricep muscles onto the thighbone and then move them up the thighbone in the standing poses (as described in chapter 5), weight

is brought to bear on the thighbones, which stimulates growth and promotes strength.

The following sequence for hypomenorrhea is to be practiced in four stages so you can build strength gradually and systematically. If your cycle has been artificially scheduled by the birth control pill, causing the menstrual flow to become light, this sequence will not bring it back to normal right away. It often takes as long as two years after coming off the pill for normal cycles to resume. Work with these four practices anyway, because they will support the system as it gradually returns to balance.

In fact, this method of practice will benefit most beginners to yoga, whether they have hypomenorrhoea or not, because it includes a wide variety of poses that put the body through its full range of motion.

PRACTICE 1: Begin by practicing all the poses in section I. Then skip to section VII to rest.

PRACTICE 2: After a few weeks or more practicing section I, gradually introduce yourself to the standing poses in section II, one or two at a time. Eventually, as you gain both physical strength and a firm understanding of these postures, you can fold them all into your practice. The standing forward extensions—Uttanasana, Parsvottanasana, and Prasarita Padottanasana—reduce toughness and tension in the abdomen. They help boost circulation in the pelvis, strengthen the internal reproductive organs, and help the glands to function properly during menstruation. They also help relieve constipation. The other standing poses in this sequence tone the abdominal organs and, similarly, strengthen the reproductive system. If you are constipated, practice them with the support of the wall to avoid further dehydration, and avoid Parivrtta Trikonasana. Complete your practice with section VII, to rest.

PRACTICE 3: Now it is time to investigate Salamba Sarvangasana I and II and its variations (section V). The inversions improve elimination and restore health and balance to the endocrine system. Halasana is particularly beneficial if the ovaries or the fallopian tubes are inactive. At the same time, you can include the seated forward bends in section VI, which release abdominal tension, stimulate the ovaries, and counteract dryness, whether manifesting as insufficient menstrual flow, or constipation. In summary, practice the entire sequence, except for section III and IV.

PRACTICE 4: When you are strong enough, add Salamba Sirsasana (section III) and the back bends (section IV) to your practice. Work with a teacher on these if you can, but also observe for yourself how each pose makes you feel and of course watch how your menstrual cycle responds. A stage 4 practice looks like this: all of section I; from section II, Utthita Trikonasana, Parsvottanasana, Parivrtta Trikonasana, Adho Mukha Vrksasana, Virabhadrasana I; all of section III; all of section IV; all of section V; section VII to rest. You may not see results overnight, but consistent practice will eventually encourage the buildup of endometrial tissue each month and allow for a healthy menstrual flow.

Do not practice these sequences during menstruation itself. Always follow menstruation with the recovery sequence in chapter 13, *no matter how light your period was.*

Practice time: 60–90 minutes

I: To Begin the Training and Set the Tone

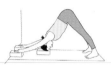

6.9c
Adho Mukha Virasana
30–60 seconds

5.5g
Adho Mukha Svanasana
with Head Support
30–60 seconds

5.4b
Uttanasana
raise head, look up
10–20 seconds

5.4h
Uttanasana with Head
Support
30–60 seconds

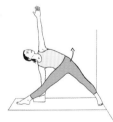

5.1d
Tadasana
20–30 seconds

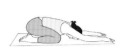

5.3a
Tadasana Urdhva Hastasana
10–20 seconds

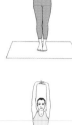

5.2c
Tadasana Urdhva
Baddhangullyasana
10–20 seconds, each side

5.8d
Utthita Hasta Padasana
20–30 seconds

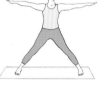

5.9a
Parsva Hasta Padasana
20–30 seconds

II: To Tone the Reproductive Organs and Build Strength

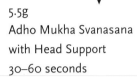

5.9d
Utthita Trikonasana with Back
Foot Against Wall
20–30 seconds, each side

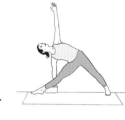

or, if constipated
5.9h
Utthita Trikonasana
with Wall and Block
20–30 seconds, each side

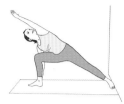

5.10h
Utthita Parsvakonasana with
Back Foot Against Wall
20–30 seconds, each side

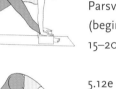

or, if constipated
5.10i
Utthita Parsvakonasana with
Back Against Wall
20–30 seconds, each side

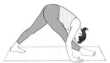

5.12d
Parsvottasana
15-20 seconds, each side, or

5.12f
Parsvottanasana with Blocks
(beginning practice)
15–20 seconds, each side

5.12e
Parsvottanasana
15–20 seconds, each side

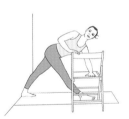

5.14d
Parivrtta Trikonasana
with Wall and Chair
(not if constipated;
beginning practice)
20–30 seconds, each side

or
5.14e
Parivrtta Trikonasana
with Wall and Block
(not if constipated)
20–30 seconds, each side

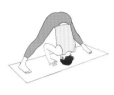

5.15d
Prasarita Padottanasana
20–30 seconds

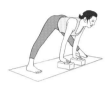

5.15e
Prasarita Padottanasana
with Hands on Blocks
1 minute

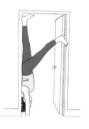

9.1h
Adho Mukha Vrksasana
in Doorway
20–30 seconds

5.4g
Uttanasana with Arms Folded
1 minute

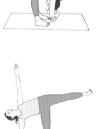

5.11e
Ardha Chandrasana
15–20 seconds, each side

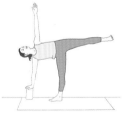

or, if constipated
5.11h
Ardha Chandrasana
against Wall
15–20 seconds, each side

III: To Improve Elimination and Reduce Tension

5.4h
Uttanasana
with Head Support
1 minute

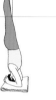

9.2d
Salamba Sirsasana
(continuing practice)
1–5 minutes

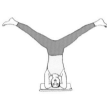

9.2g
Upavistha Konasana
in Salamba Sirsasana
(continuing practice)
20–30 seconds

9.2h
Baddha Konasana
in Salamba Sirsasana
(continuing practice)
20–30 seconds
or

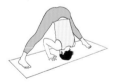

5.15d
Prasarita Padottanasana
(beginning practice)
1 minute

IV: To Energize and Strengthen the Pelvic Muscles

Do not practice these poses when constipated.

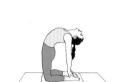

10.1e
Ustrasana
(continuing practice)
20–30 seconds

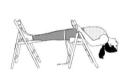

10.2d
Viparita Dandasana II
(continuing practice)
30–60 seconds, increasing
to 5 minutes with practice
or

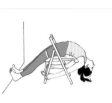

10.2h
Viparita Dandasana II
with Two Chairs
(beginning practice)
20–30 seconds

6.17a
Supported Bharadvajasana II
20–30 seconds, each side

V: To Promote Feelings of Peace and Well-Being

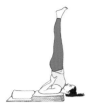

9.3f
Salamba Sarvangasana I
2–5 minutes,
increasing with practice

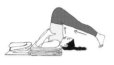

9.6b
Halasana
1–5 minutes

9.6g
Supta Konasana
30–60 seconds

9.7a
Parsva Halasana
15–20 seconds, each side

Or, If Tired

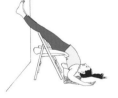

9.4e
Salamba Sarvangasana II
3–5 minutes

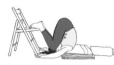

9.5c
Karnapidasana with Chair
20–30 seconds

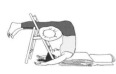

9.8e
Ardha Halasana with
Thighs Raised on Bolster
3–5 minutes

VI: To Alleviate Tension and Relieve Constipation

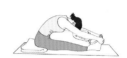

6.9e
Adho Mukha Virasana
with Bolster
30–60 seconds

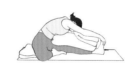

7.4f
Paschimottanasana
with Vertical Bolster
20–30 seconds

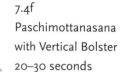

6.12a
Adho Mukha Swastikasana
(beginning practice)
30–60 seconds,
change legs, 30–60 seconds

7.1l
Janu Sirsasana
with Vertical Bolster
and Blankets
20–30 seconds, each side

7.4f
Paschimottanasana
with Vertical Bolster
3–5 minutes

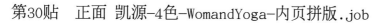

第30贴　正面　凯源-4色-WomandYoga-内页拼版.job

VII: To Rest

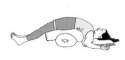

8.10d
Setu Bandha Sarvangasana II
over Crossed Bolsters
3–8 minutes

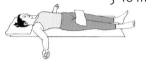

8.14e
Savasana with Sandbag
5–10 minutes

22

Absence of Menstruation: Getting Back to Normal

AMENORRHEA, the absence of periods, is divided into two types: primary and secondary. Primary amenorrhea, which is when menstruation never starts, is very rare. Secondary amenorrhea is the absence of menstrual periods for six months in a woman who was previously regular or for twelve months in a woman who had irregular periods.

Amenorrhea should not to be confused with oligomenorrhea, which refers to infrequent periods, that is, having fewer than eight periods a year. Menopausal women and adolescent girls commonly experience oligomenorrhea.

This may seem obvious, but it must be stated: if your periods have stopped, get a pregnancy test! The most common reason for the cessation of periods is pregnancy.

Other reasons for failure to menstruate include trauma or stress, obsessive dieting, excessive exercising, and occasionally a glandular disorder, such as polycystic ovary syndrome (PCOS), Cushing's disease (overactive adrenal glands), hypothyroidism (underactive thyroid gland), or a cyst on the hypothalamus or pituitary gland. Some medications can cause amenorrhea, as can some surgeries, such as dilation and curettage (commonly called a D & C, a scraping of the lining of the uterus) or cervical conization (the removal of tissue from the cervix).

You can see from this list that if menstruation stops, it is important to find out why, because amenorrhea may be a symptom of a serious condition. Even if the problem is functional amenorrhea (cessation of periods with no disease present), it is most important to get the cycle going again, because this condition can lead to other problems, such as loss of bone density, infertility, and the early onset of menopause.

The absence of menstruation also means that ovulation has failed to occur. Menstruation and ovulation are related to body weight. Girls begin to menstruate once they achieve a critical weight, and if body weight drops too low, menstruation stops. A woman's body is genetically programmed to protect her reproductive capacity. It is wrapped in a layer of subcutaneous fat so that she can feed her young during periods of deprivation. If this layer of fat gets too thin (as with anorexia and excess exercise) or too thick (as with PCOS), it affects the healthy functioning of the hormonal system. Several factors contribute to polycystic ovary syndrome. One of the most significant is a diet high in sugar and refined carbohydrates. Another major cause, according to John R. Lee, M.D., is exposure of female embryos to environmental pollutants. These xenobiotics act like estrogen on the developing baby's tissues, causing the ovarian follicles to be dysfunctional.

This damage, says Dr. Lee, is not apparent until after puberty.

Ovarian cysts can also be exacerbated by stress. The hypothalamus gland plays a particularly important role here. It is a crucial part of a chain reaction of hormones that triggers the ovary to release an egg, thus beginning the process that will lead to a period two weeks later. Some clinicians have hypothesized that the hypothalamus is directly affected by emotional and psychological factors. Emotional trauma, such as intense fright, grief, loss, anger, or excessive anxiety, may disturb the sensitive feedback system that operates between the pituitary, the hypothalamus, the adrenals, and the ovaries, causing estrogen levels to drop and the period to slow down or stop altogether.

These days the most common causes for amenorrhea are dieting and overexercising. The syndrome known as the female athletic triad, which mostly affects dancers and athletes, is a condition in which menstruation has either ceased or failed to start due to eating disorders, excessive exercise, or a combination of the two. This dangerous condition can result in bone loss and eventually in osteoporosis. Bone development is intricately tied to healthy hormonal functioning, which in a female past the age of puberty means having regular periods. Jordon D. Metzl, a physician at the Hospital for Special Surgery, in New York, says that failure to support healthy bone growth is especially harmful for adolescent girls, because bone development only happens until age thirty, after which bone mass is gradually lost. In one study, women aged thirty-five who missed ovulation one or more times a year had an average loss of 4 percent of their bone density over a year.

If your periods have stopped due to low calorie intake, increase your food consumption and include plenty of calcium-rich foods, such as dark leafy greens, nut milks, milk, vegetable and fruit juices, and legumes. Whole-foods educator Roberta Atti informed me that women who exercise compulsively often have imbalanced diets where certain food groups have been eliminated. Make sure your diet includes all the whole food groups.

Practice

When hormone levels have been thrown off balance, either by excessive physical exercise or an eating disorder or both, and menstruation has ceased, do not practice the following sequence, as it will further deplete energy and strength. It is time to rest. Go easy on the body and avoid energetic exercise until the cycle is back to normal. Practice the restorative sequence in chapter 14 until menstruation shows signs of returning. Then follow the guidelines in this chapter.

Similarly, if the absence of menstruation is caused by hyperthyroidism (overactive thyroid), do not practice the following sequence. Although a malfunctioning thyroid responds very well to yoga, it is necessary to practice with the guidance of a competent yoga teacher. The following sequence is not appropriate for women with PCOS or Cushing's disease or any other organic disease.

When the body stops functioning in some way, especially when the reproductive system is involved, there has often been a preceding emotional difficulty. The cure for menstrual malfunction goes hand in hand with the relief of emotional depression. Geeta S. Iyengar, author of *Yoga: A Gem for Women*, recommends back bends, twists, and inversions to get the menstrual cycle going when it has been disturbed as a result of emotional distress. The following practice sequence emphasizes back bends, which open the heart center, release emotional blockages, and help dispel gloom and grief.

Surya Namaskara (see also chapter 5) in section I is an energetic flowing set of asana that helps take your attention outward. Alternatively, you can warm up at the beginning of your session by practicing these poses individually, that is, without jumping between them. This is especially recommended for those with joint or back problems. Beginners can start by first learning to jump between Uttanasana and Adho Mukha Svanasana only.

Jump rhythmically from pose to pose and use your breath (take one or two normal breaths during each pose) to time them. To help you get into the swing of it, I have indicated which breath goes with which movement. Make them easy breaths, not too long and not too short.

Section II helps to build strength and reduce stress. The inversions in section III and IV nourish the glands with a good supply of blood. Taken together, they have a stabilizing effect on hormonal activity and the nervous system. Women should practice the inversions every day of the postmenstrual phase and at least twice a week when not menstruating. Bharadvajasana, in section IV, massages, stimulates, and strengthens the internal reproductive organs. It also prepares the spine and torso for back bends.

Backbends, which are also in section IV, are the heart of this sequence. They stimulate the pituitary, pineal, and thyroid glands. They also strengthen the pelvic organs and stimulate the ovaries and adrenal glands. Although back bends are an important factor in bringing hormonal activity to life, beginning students should be cautious. Begin by building strength with the standing poses (if possible with a teacher) before attempting back bends. You can also work on other standing poses not included in this chapter, by following the guidelines in chapter 5. (When menstruation is arrested due to depression or trauma, avoid the forward bends.) Introduce yourself to the back bends gradually, beginning with Viparita Dandasana II. Thereafter practice this pose to warm up the spine in preparation for the other back bends. Ustrasana is the next back bend to learn; make sure you are thoroughly familiar with it before moving on to Urdhva Danurasana. Along with Kapotasana and Supta Baddha Konasana in Viparita Dandasana II (you need only practice one or the other in a session), Urdhva Danurasana is a strenuous pose and is not suitable for beginning students.

Practice time: 60–90 minutes

I: To Reduce Nervous Energy and Warm Up: Surya Namaskara

5.1d
Tadasana
Inhale and swing
your arms up into

5.3a
Tadasana Urdhva Hastasana
With an exhalation,
sweep forward
and down into

5.4c
Uttanasana
With an inhalation,
pull forward
and up into

5.4b
Uttanasana
Raise your head and
with an exhalation
jump back into

5.5d
Adho Mukha Svanasana
With an inhalation
swing forward
and up into

5.6c
Urdhva Mukha Svanasana
With an exhalation,
drop down into

5.7d
Chatturanga Dandasana
With an inhalation,
push up into

5.6c
Urdhva Mukha Svanasana
With an exhalation,
swing back into

5.5d
Adho Mukha Svanasana
Exhale and jump forward into

5.4c
Uttanasana
Inhaling, swing your arms
up into

5.1d
Tadasana

Repeat the cycle 3 times.
Omit Tadasana on the way
through, but return to it
as the final pose,
for 20–30 seconds.

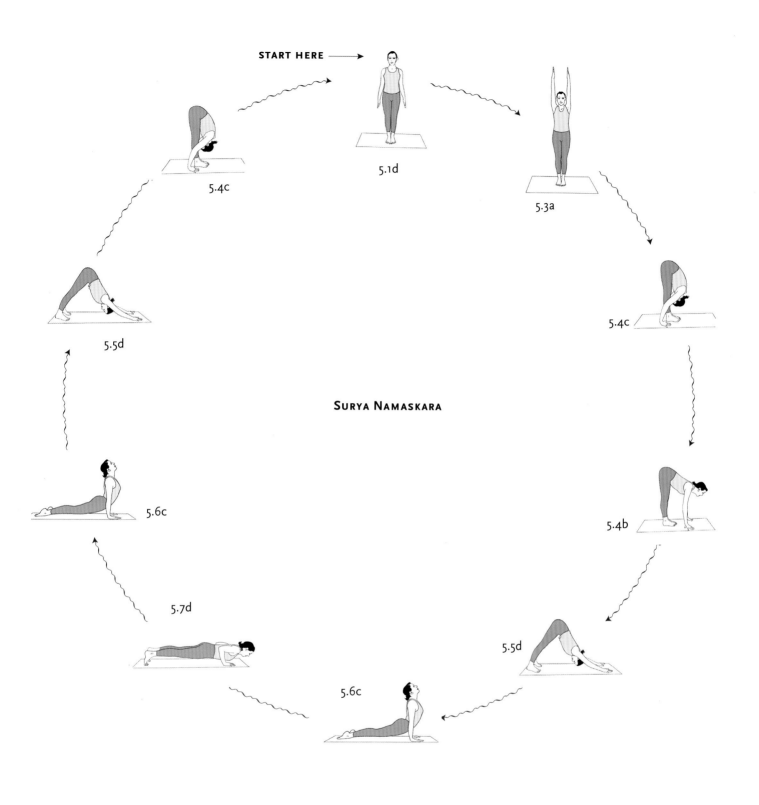

START HERE →

5.1d

5.3a

5.4c

5.4c

5.4b

SURYA NAMASKARA

5.5d

5.5d

5.6c

5.6c

5.7d

II: To Build Strength and Reduce Stress   **III: For a Positive Outlook**

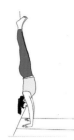

9.1d
Adho Mukha Vrksasana
20–30 seconds

5.4h
Uttanasana with Head
Support
1 minute

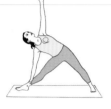

5.9c
Utthita Trikonasana
20–30 seconds, each side

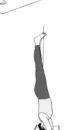

5.15d
Prasarita Padottanasana
1 minute

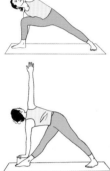

5.10g
Utthita Parsvakonasana
20–30 seconds, each side

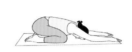

9.2d
Salamba Sirsasana
1–5 minutes

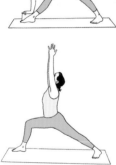

5.14c
Parivrtta Trikonasana
20–30 seconds, each side

6.9c
Adho Mukha Virasana
20–30 seconds

5.13d
Virabhadrasana I
20–30 seconds, each side

IV: To Open the Chest and Lift the Spirits

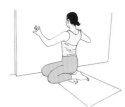

6.15c
Bharadvajasana
20–30 seconds, each side

10.2d
Viparita Dandasana II
(continuing practice)
30–60 seconds, increasing to
5 minutes with practice

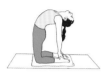

10.1e
Ustrasana
20–30 seconds, 1–3 times

10.4f
Urdhva Dhanurasana
(continuing practice)
5–10 seconds, 1–6 times

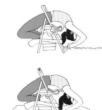

10.5c or 10.5d
Kapotasana
(advanced practice)
30–60 seconds, increasing
to 3 minutes with practice
or

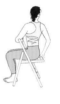

10.3d or 10.3e
Supta Baddha Konasana
in Viparita Dandasana II
(advanced practice)
30–60 seconds, increasing
to 5 minutes with practice

6.17a
Supported Bharadvajasana II
20–30 seconds, each side

5.4l
Parsva Uttanasana with Wall
20–30 seconds, 2 times

第32贴　正面 凯源-4色-WomandYoga-内页拼版.job

V: To Calm the Mind and Cool Down

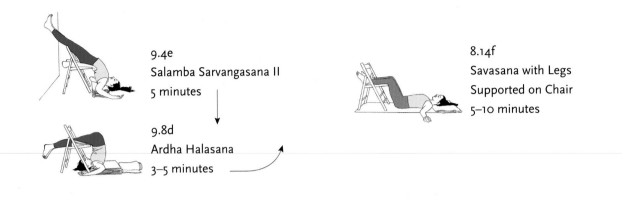

9.4e
Salamba Sarvangasana II
5 minutes

9.8d
Ardha Halasana
3–5 minutes

8.14f
Savasana with Legs
Supported on Chair
5–10 minutes

第32贴　反面　凯源-4色-WomandYoga-内页拼版.job

23

Irregular Menstruation: Reestablishing the Rhythm

A REGULARLY RECURRING menstrual cycle is a good indicator of a woman's overall health and well-being. By the same token, bleeding that occurs outside the normal pattern may be your body's way of telling you that all is not as it should be.

But what is a normal pattern? While the common assumption that menstruation should occur at exactly twenty-eight-day intervals reflects the possibility that we are connected to the seasons of the moon, only 12.4 percent of women have twenty-eight-day cycles. Most cycles are between twenty-three and thirty-five days, and this is considered, at least by orthodox medicine, to be healthy. Orthodox medicine also considers it normal when women's cycles vary from month to month. Menstruation can be considered irregular when bleeding occurs outside of your normal pattern, or when you miss periods more than occasionally.

Irregular periods are most common in the first three years following menarche (the onset of menstruation) and during perimenopause (the years preceding menopause). At other times during a woman's life, menstrual irregularity can be caused by a variety of factors and should be always checked out by a doctor, even if you are perimenopausal, to rule out organic causes. These can include pelvic or cervical lesions, infec-

tions or inflammations, benign growths such as fibroids or polyps, ovarian cysts, polycystic ovary syndrome, or precancerous conditions. Another cause could be problems with an IUD (intrauterine device). Where irregular menstruation is not caused by an organic abnormality, anovulation (the absence of ovulation or infrequent ovulation) is usually the cause. Anovulation occurs when the body does not receive the necessary stimulus to release an egg, and the subsequent release of estrogen and progesterone fails to take place as it should.

Inadequate ovarian function can have many underlying causes. Some clinicians suggest that lack of regular exposure to sunlight (and therefore the absence of adequate amounts of vitamin D) contributes to menstrual irregularity. Certainly we are now exposed to less natural darkness and less natural daylight than in times past. According to Native American lore, an irregular or malfunctioning menstrual cycle can be corrected if a woman sleeps out under the light of the full moon. In societies that did not use artificial sources of light, moonlight may have had a more powerful effect on women's systems and may have triggered ovulation. Air travel also disturbs circadian rhythms and is a notorious disrupter of women's periods.

Other possible factors that could upset the delicate interplay between brain, ovaries, and uterus include excess body fat or sudden weight loss, certain medications (sleeping pills, tranquilizers, antidepressants, narcotics), overexercise (interpreted by the body as stress), and some herbs, such as ginseng. Low thyroid function and pituitary dysfunction can also cause irregular periods. In the two years after women stop taking birth control pills, they are five times more likely to complain of infrequent or irregular periods. Additionally, an illness (and possibly a fever) that occurs before ovulation may cause ovulation (and therefore menstruation) to be either delayed or skipped altogether.

A stressful lifestyle may also disrupt hormone balance. Bouts of severe anxiety or depression can change the balance of neurotransmitters in the brain and affect hypothalamic function, especially where it is associated with emotional disturbances arising out of family issues. Often such cycles are accompanied by a heavy flow. The woman whose cycles are sensitive to stress may also find that when she assumes responsibilities at the expense of her innermost emotional needs, she pays a toll with her health.

Since anovulatory cycles are associated with osteoporosis and infertility, it is important to preserve hormonal balance. A recent study found that women with irregular menstruation have a greater chance of developing rheumatoid arthritis later in life. Women from ancient cultures, who understood the importance of a regular menstrual cycle, had some wonderful customs. Australian aboriginal women made a cat's cradle, forming a pattern of three entwined and interconnecting links, said to represent the menstrual blood of three women, as part of a ritualized visualization process to synchronize their cycles with each other. In the West we now know that our men-

strual cycles respond to each other's pheromones.

When stress causes menstruation to be irregular, how does a woman remedy the situation without resorting to drugs or invasive hormone therapy?

Start by keeping a journal for three to four months to get a clear idea of what is happening, so you can organize your practice around your individual cycle. What is your usual pattern of menstruation? How has it changed? True menstruation is that which occurs between twelve to sixteen days following the release of an egg. The quality of the flow should be fairly consistent from month to month. Any other occurrence of bleeding is either anovulatory, normal midcycle spotting, or symptomatic of an organic problem.

Yoga is an effective way of reducing the effects of stress on the body–mind and restoring hormonal balance.

Practice

There are three golden rules for dealing with irregular or unusual bleeding:

1. Always practice one of the menstrual sequences in this book during the cleansing (active bleeding) phase of your cycle. Select one that is appropriate to your needs. A menstrual sequence will rest you and will minimize the stress that may be contributing to irregularity.

2. Always practice the postmenstrual sequence when your period is over (see chapter 13), whether it was preceded by ovulation or not. The postmenstrual sequence, which is composed mostly of inverted poses, helps establish a healthy hormonal rhythm. Salamba Sirsasana stimulates the master gland, the pituitary. The pituitary releases the hormones that begin the process of maturing the follicles in your ovaries, so that

estrogen, which is necessary for ovulation, begins to build. Salamba Sarvangasana II, Halasana, Setu Bandha Sarvangasana I, and Setu Bandha Sarvangasana II balance the effect Salamba Sirsasana has on the pituitary gland, regulate thyroid output, and cool and calm the system. Taken together, the inversions and their variations help the nervous system and the uterus recover from menstruation and set the rhythm for future cycles.

3. When the menstrual and postmenstrual phases are over, make sure your yoga practice reflects your emotional and physical needs, so that you relieve stress. If irregular periods are combined with an excessive or heavy flow, follow the guidelines in chapter 20 throughout the rest of the month. Otherwise organize your practice to include a wide range of poses throughout the month. One way to do this is to be methodical. Once the postmenstrual phase is over, begin by introducing the standing poses into your practice, and make them the main focus of your yoga for a week. Practice Utthita Trikonasana and Ardha Chandrasana Facing Wall if irregularity is caused by organic problems. Then introduce the forward bends and twists, and make them the main focus of your practice for a week. Do the inverted poses regularly (every day if possible) throughout the month. By ovulation, when the body and mind are at their most energetic, you should be including all the postures that you have in your repertoire, including the back bends. Practice back bends sensitively and carefully however, especially if your cycle is erratic. And don't just practice them on their own; include a variety of other poses in each session. Toward the end of your cycle, practice the sequence given in this chapter. Practice pranayama regularly, throughout the month.

Delayed Menstruation

When stress affects the cycle, menstruation is more likely to be delayed than speeded up. Remember, though, it is delayed ovulation that is delaying your period. Once you have ovulated, the course of action is determined; you will menstruate about twelve to sixteen days later. (For most women, the length of time from ovulation to the onset of bleeding doesn't vary by more than a day or two.) Therefore, when menstruation is delayed, it is unlikely that you will be able to "bring on" your period. Practice the sequence recommended in this chapter, which includes inversions to balance hormones and seated forward bends to reduce tension.

Spotting Before Your Period

Sometimes a woman can spot for five to ten days before her period starts, and the blood can be dark, grayish, or almost black in color. (If this occurs, see a physician to rule out thyroid problems, fibroids, endometriosis, or endometrial polyps.) In the same category as spotting is the period that appears to start and then disappears for a few days. For both of these situations, practice the forward bends: Adho Mukha Virasana, Adho Mukha Svanasana, Uttanasana, Janu Sirsasana, and Paschimottanasana. Support the head, to reduce hardness and tension in the abdomen and to boost oxygen to the ovaries. *Do not* practice any back bends or reclining poses— not even Setu Bandha Sarvangasana I or II. However, if your period returns with fatigue or any kind of stress, such as a heavy flow or cramping, then practice the (three) reclining poses in the restorative sequence described in chapter 14, which *does* include Setu Bandha Sarvangasana II, and finish with Savasana. Avoid the inversions when you are spotting, because they will further disturb the menstrual flow.

Midcycle Spotting

If you are experiencing normal midcycle spotting, this should not be a cause for alarm. It is caused by the sudden decrease in the amount of available estrogen, and it occurs mostly among women who are on the pill. It is fine to practice inversions at this time.

Spotting After Your Period

If you spot after your period, hold off on the inversions until all residue of menstrual flow has stopped. Practice the reclining poses—Supta Baddha Konasana, Supta Virasana, Matsyasana or Supta Swastikasana, and Setu Bandha Sarvangasana II—until the flow stops completely.

Missed Periods

The occasionally missed period requires no specific treatment. Provided it is not due to menopause or pregnancy, you have probably failed to ovulate that month. If you are skipping periods a lot, it may be due to stress, inadequate diet, over-exercise, or depletion (see chapter 22). In a month where you fail to menstruate, practice the menstrual sequence anyway (see chapter 12) around the time you would have menstruated. Follow this with the postmenstrual sequence.

Irregular Periods
Caused by Organic Abnormalities

When irregular or unusual bleeding is due to organic abnormalities (ovarian cysts and the like),

hormone imbalance and stress may be the underlying cause. The guidelines in this chapter can still be applied. Consult an experienced teacher for poses to support any medical procedure you may decide upon. Similarly, if you are perimenopausal and your symptoms are similar to those mentioned, you can still honor your cyclic nature. Navigate around perimenopausal menstrual irregularities to minimize discomfort in a similar manner.

When Your Period Is Early

When your cycles are speeded up, check that you have calculated the length of your cycle correctly. If the length of the cycle is taken from the end of the period to the beginning of the next, the cycle appears to be short. Calculate the length of the cycle from the first day of bleeding to the day before you begin to bleed again. If you spot for a few days prior to your period, do not include that in your calculations. The first day of the cycle is considered to be the first full day of menstrual flow, even if it is light (which is the case for many women). Rule out the possibility that you are having an unusually long cycle and then having breakthrough bleeding. This is sometimes mistaken for normal menstruation, so you need to determine whether ovulation has taken place or not. If bleeding is preceded by premenstrual mood changes, bloating, breast tenderness, and maybe some degree of dysmenorrhea, you have probably ovulated. However, when periods come out of the blue or your cycle is erratic, and the flow is either unusually heavy or light, it often means that the delicate interplay between estrogen and progesterone has been thrown off balance and you haven't ovulated.

Although it is not possible to prescribe a one-fits-all yoga sequence, these postures will help relieve anxiety and restore hormone balance. If you can predict approximately when your period is likely to happen, practice this sequence for the eight to ten days prior to menstruation (postovulation) as part of the process of restoring balance.

Practice time: 60–90 minutes

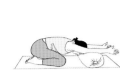

6.9e
Adho Mukha Virasana with Bolster
30–60 seconds

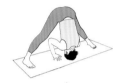

5.5g
Adho Mukha Svanasana with Head Support
30–60 seconds

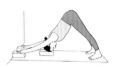

5.4h
Uttanasana with Head Support
1 minute

5.15d
Prasarita Padottanasana
1 minute

9.2d
Salamba Sirsasana
1–5 minutes

II: To Reduce Anxiety and Stimulate Circulation in the Pelvis and Chest

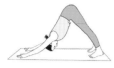

5.5d
Adho Mukha Svanasana
30–60 seconds

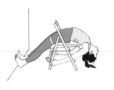

10.2d
Viparita Dandasana II
30–60 seconds, increasing to
5 minutes with practice

6.17a
Supported Bharadvajasana II
20–30 seconds, each side

III: To Keep Ovaries Healthy and Promote a Regular Menstrual Cycle

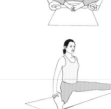

6.2d
Baddha Konasana
with Rolled Blankets
1–5 minutes

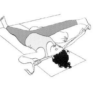

6.3a
Upavistha Konasana
1–2 minutes

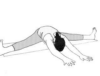

8.13c
Supta Padangusthasana II
with Bolster
20–30 seconds

IV: To Dissolve Abdominal Tension and Quiet the Brain

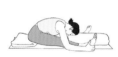

7.4g
Paschimottanasa
with Legs Apart and Bolster
20–30 seconds

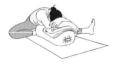

7.1m
Janu Sirsasana with Legs
Apart and Head Support
30–60 seconds, 2 times

6.5b
Adho Mukha Upavistha
Konasana
30–60 seconds

7.4h
Paschimottanasana
with Legs Apart
3–5 minutes

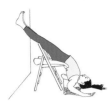

9.4e
Salamba Sarvangasana II
3–5 minutes

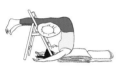

9.4f
Viparita Karani in Salamba
Sarvangasana on Chair
30–60 seconds

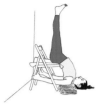

9.4g
Baddha Konasana in Salamba
Sarvangasana on Chair
30–60 seconds

9.8d
Ardha Halasana
3–5 minutes ⟶

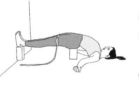

8.9c
Setu Bandha Sarvangasana I
(continuing practice)
or

8.10a
Setu Bandha Sarvangasana II
(beginning practice)
3–8 minutes

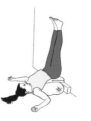

9.9d
Viparita Karani
5–10 minutes

8.14d
Savasana
5–10 minutes

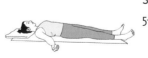

Resources

Books

Clennell, Bobby. *A Cosmic Body Map.*
    Available from www.toolsforyoga.net
————. *Iyengar Yoga Glossary.*
    Available from www.toolsforyoga.net
    www.customyogaprops.com
    www.yogamatters.com
————. *Props and Ailments.*
    Available from www.toolsforyoga.net
    www.customyogaprops.com
    www.unitywoods.com • www.yogamatters.com
    www.yogaprops@jvana.de
Iyengar, B. K. S. *Light on Life: The Yoga Journey to Wholeness, Inner Peace, and Ultimate Freedom.* Emmaus, PA: Rodale, 2005.
————. *Light on Yoga.* New York: Schocken Books, 1995.
————. *Light on Pranayama: The Yogic Art of Breathing.* New York: Crossroad, 1985.
————. *Light on the Yoga Sutras of Patanjali.* New York: Thorsons, 2003.
————. *Tree of Yoga.* Boston: Shambhala, 2002.
————. *Yoga: The Path to Holistic Health.* New York: Dorling Kindersley, 2001.
Iyengar, Geeta S. *Yoga: A Gem for Women.* Toronto: Timeless Books, 2002.

Journal

Namarupa: Categories of Indian Thought
www.namarupa.org

Props

Tools for Yoga
www.toolsforyoga.net (including the Pune Belt)

Iyengar Yoga

For information about Iyengar Yoga, classes, and certified teachers, contact the Iyengar Yoga National Association of the United States, www.iynaus.org.

From the Publisher

RODMELL PRESS publishes books on yoga, Buddhism, aikido, and Taoism. In the Bhagavadgita it is written, "Yoga is skill in action." It is our hope that our books will help individuals develop a more skillful practice—one that brings peace to their daily lives and to the earth.

We thank those whose support, encouragement, and practical advise sustain us in our efforts. In particular, we are grateful to Reb Anderson, B. K. S. Iyengar, Wendy Palmer, and Yvonne Rand for their inspiration.

To request a catalog or receive e-announcements about new titles, contact us at:
    (510) 841-3123 or (800) 841-3123
    (510) 841-3123 (fax)
    info@rodmellpress.com • www.rodmellpress.com

Rodmell Press is distributed by Publishers Group West:
    (800) 788-3123 • (510) 528-5511 (sales fax)
    info@pgw.com

About the Author

BOBBY CLENNELL has been teaching Iyengar Yoga for over thirty years. She is a core faculty member of the Iyengar Yoga Institute of New York, where she teaches five classes a week, including the women's class and the prenatal class. She also teaches workshops throughout the United States and Europe and leads retreats in the United Kingdom, Tobago, and Mexico, with her husband, yoga teacher Lindsey Clennell.

Bobby began practicing yoga in London in the early 1970s, while working as a costume designer and animator. In 1976, Bobby (along with Lindsey and sons Miles and Jake), made her first trip to study with B. K. S. Iyengar in Pune, India. She has returned every two years to continue her study. She was given an Iyengar Yoga teaching certificate in 1977.

In the 1980s, Bobby's interest in women's issues was sparked by her studies with Mr. Iyengar's daughter, Geeta Iyengar. While Mr. Iyengar was teaching the main class, the women who were menstruating were sent to the back of the room to work more quietly. Geeta showed these women how. This experience awakened Bobby to the need for a woman's yoga practice, and it has been the focus of her teaching ever since.

She is the creator of a short film, entitled "Yantra," based on the movements of B.K.S. Iyengar during his own asana practice.

Bobby Clennell lives in New York City. For more information about her teaching schedule and film, visit www.bobbyclennell.com.

Index

hypomenorrhea. *See* scanty periods
hypothyroidism, 212, 219

immune system, boosting, 99, 121, 144, 189
Indian traditions, 6. *See also* ayurveda
infrequent periods, 219
insomnia
    amount of sleep needed, 191
    avoiding Tadasana Urdhva Bad-
        dhangullyasana, 33
    ayurveda on, 192
    dream deprivation from, 191–192
    good sleep habits, 192
    head wrapping for relieving, 100
    hormonal fluctuations and, 191
    poses relieving, 111, 121
    practice, 192–193
    pranayama alternatives for, 151–152
    sequences, 193–195
Interrupted Inhalation, Normal Exhalation.
    See Viloma I
inverted poses. *See also specific poses*
    Adho Mukha Vrksasana, 122–123
    Ardha Halasana, 128, 136–138
    avoiding during period, 18–19, 162
    benefits in general, 121
    cautions in general, 121
    Halasana, 133–134
    Karnapidasana, 133
    Parsva Halasana, 136
    Salamba Sarvangasana I, 125, 127–130
    Salamba Sarvangasana II, 125, 131–132
    Salamba Sirsasana, 124–126
    Supta Konasana, 134–135
    Viparita Karani, 132, 138
Inverted Relaxation Pose. *See* Viparita Karani
Inverted Staff Pose. *See* Viparita Dandasana II
irregular periods
    causes of, 16, 227–228, 230
    delayed, 229
    early, 230–231
    golden rules for, 228–229
    midcycle spotting, 230
    missed periods, 230
    from organic abnormalities, 227–228, 230
    poses counteracting, 55, 87, 88, 144
    practice, 228–231
    spotting after period, 230
    spotting before period, 229–230
irritability. *See* tension or stress
Is Menstruation Obsolete?, 7
Iyengar, B. K. S., 2, 15–16, 198, 234
Iyengar, Geeta S.
    author's study with, 2, 16
    foreword by, xi–xii
    on menstrual energy as heat, 6
    on postmenstrual phase, 11–12
    on restarting the menstrual cycle, 220
    on shoulder work during menstruation, 72
    on Supta Virasana, 104
    on twists, 61
    Yoga: A Gem for Women, 2, 61, 104,
        220, 234
Iyengar, Prashant, 2

Iyengar Yoga
    development of, 15
    further information, 234
    standing poses as basis of, 31
    vocabulary of, 29
Iyengar Yoga Glossary, 234

Janu Sirsasana
    benefits, 88
    with Blankets and Strap, 90
    cautions, 89
    with Chair, 90, 91
    with Horizontal Bolster, 90, 91, 164, 182,
        183, 194, 202
    with Legs Apart, 90–91, 207, 210
    with Legs Apart and Head Support, 232
    practice, 89
    with Rolled Blanket, 90
    with Rolled Blanket, Washcloth, and
        Block, 90
    in sequences, 164, 168, 182, 183, 188,
        194, 202, 207, 210, 217, 232
    with Vertical Bolster and Blankets, 90, 91,
        202, 217
Judaism, Orthodox, 5, 6
Jumping from Tadasana to Utthita Hasta
    Padasana, 42–43

Kapotasana, 148–149, 225
Karnapidasana, 133, 217
kidneys, poses toning, 63, 64, 111
knee problems
    cautions for poses
        Ardha Chandrasana, 49
        Matsyasana, 107
        Padmasana, 82, 107
        sitting poses and twists, 61–62
        Supta Virasana, 105
        Triang Mukhaikapada Paschimot-
            tanasana, 92
        Virasana, 74
    poses to avoid
        Ardha Padma Paschimottanasana, 94
        Bharadvajasana, 83
        jumping, 42, 58
        Parsva Adho Mukha Swastikasana, 80
        Surya Namaskara, 58
Kneeling Cow Face Pose. *See*
    Gomukhasana in Vajrasana
Kneeling Prayer Pose. *See* Paschima
    Namaskarasana in Vajrasana

late period, 229. *See also* irregular periods
Lateral Plow Pose. *See* Parsva Halasana
Lawler, Robert, 5
Lee, John R., 219–220
leukorrhea, 64, 68
lifting spirits, sequences for, 171, 225
Light on Life, 234
Light on Pranayama, 234
Light on the Yoga Sutras of Patanjali, 234
Light on Yoga, 2, 15, 234
liver, 61, 91
longevity, inverted poses for, 121

Lotus Pose. *See* Padmasana
low blood pressure
    cautions for poses, 33, 99
    poses benefiting, 56, 103
    poses to avoid, 35, 56
Lu, Nan, 6
luteal phase of menstrual cycle, 12, 19–20,
    165

manic episodes, back bends and, 140
mat, nonslip, 26
Matsyasana
    overview, 106–107
    in sequences, 163, 201, 206
McClintock, Martha, 10
meditation, yoga as, 20
menarche
    earlier in modern times, 1, 9
    honoring and acknowledging, xi, 5, 10,
        161
    overview, 9–10
    word roots for, 9
menopause, 13
menorrhagia. *See* excessive or prolonged
    bleeding
menstrual cycle
    as bond to natural world, 2–3
    factors disrupting, 11
    as indicator of energetic balance, 211
    length of, 10
    as opportunity for self-awareness, 169
    phases of, 11–12, 165
    pheromones' influence on, 10
    physiology of, 11–13
    postmenstrual phase, 11–12
    practice during phases, 17–20
    synchronization of, 10–11
menstrual headaches, relieving, 37, 88. *See
    also* migraine headaches; tension
    headaches
menstruation. *See also* days after period;
    during your period; PMS (premenstrual
    syndrome)
    absence of, 219–226
    cultures of, 5–6
    excessive or prolonged bleeding, 159,
        169, 203–210
    increase in number of periods, 1, 6–7
    irregular, 227–231
    modern life and, 1–2
    neglect of, 1–2, 5
    as obsolete, 7
    reasons for, 7–8
    scanty, 54, 211–213
    start of (menarche), xi, 1, 5, 9–10, 61
Metzl, Jordon D., 220
migraine headaches. *See also* menstrual
    headaches, relieving; tension
    headaches
    avoiding Ujjayi II, 157
    avoiding Viloma I, 159
    ayurveda on, 179
    Chinese medicine on, 179–180
    as PMS symptoms, 179